EMPATH

A Survival Guide for the Highly Sensitive
Person- Achieve Emotional & Spiritual Healing

TORI DASANI

Contents

Introduction	vii
1. What is an Empath?	1
2. Are you an Empath? Self-assessment Test	15
3. Common Traits of the Empath	31
4. Empath Types	55
5. Benefits, drawbacks, and dangers of empathic power	71
6. Making the Most of it	79
7. Protecting the Empathic Self through	90
8. Staying Light	120
9. Finding Empathic Joy	138
10. Finding Peace	148
Conclusion	157

Copyright 2019 by Tori Dasani - All rights reserved.

This book is provided with the sole purpose of providing relevant information on a specific topic for which every reasonable effort has been made to ensure that it is both accurate and understandable. Nevertheless, by purchasing this book, you consent to the fact that the author, as well as the publisher, are in no way experts on the topics contained herein, regardless of any claims as such that may be made within. As such, any suggestions or recommendations that are made within are done so purely for entertainment value. It is recommended that you always consult a professional before undertaking any of the advice or techniques discussed within.

This is a legally binding declaration that is considered both valid and fair by both the Committee of Publishers Association and the American Bar Association and should be considered as legally binding within the United States.

The reproduction, transmission, and duplication of any of the content found herein, including any specific or extended information will be done as an illegal act regardless of the end form the information ultimately takes. This includes copied versions of the work physical, digital and audio unless express consent of the Publisher is provided beforehand. Any additional rights reserved.

Furthermore, the information that can be found within the pages described forthwith shall be considered both accurate and truthful when it comes to the recounting of facts. As such, any use, correct or incorrect, of the provided information will render the Publisher free of responsibility as to the actions taken outside of their direct purview. Regardless, there are zero scenarios where the original author or the Publisher can be deemed liable in any fashion for any damages or hardships that may result from any of the information discussed herein.

Additionally, the information in the following pages is intended only for informational purposes and should thus be thought of as universal. As befitting its nature, it is presented without assurance regarding its prolonged validity or interim quality. Trademarks that are mentioned are done without written consent and can in no way be considered an endorsement from the trademark holder.

Introduction

Congratulations on purchasing Empath: a Survival Guide for the Highly Sensitive Person, and thank you for doing so. Within these pages, you will find in-depth descriptions of the empathy's interior world, the traits and habits that differentiate them from the average individual, and a quiz to help you understand your degree of empathic ability. You will develop a thorough understanding of empathy as the invisible substance of emotional connection, and learn how to distinguish healthy forms of empathy from those forms that can be draining, overwhelming, or even destructive.

If you should discover that your empathy quotient is high or advanced, you'll also find many tools, practices, and guides here to help you manage intense emotions (whether they are yours or someone else's) and maintain your energy reserves, shielding your essence from psychic vampires and toxic relationship dynamics. From the realms of western medicine, neuroscience, psychology, and spiritual healing traditions, you will learn strategies for managing empathic power that can be combined and tailored to suit your individual needs. You'll be steered first towards the goal of finding joy and gratitude for your empathy, though it can indeed be challenging to manage. Secondly, your goal will be to find inner peace, a form of energetic balance that provides enough stability for you to weather whatever emotional storms life might throw at you.

There are plenty of books on this subject on the market, so thank you again for choosing this one! Every effort was made to ensure it is full of as much useful and accurate information as possible. Please enjoy!

1

What is an Empath?

The terminology we use to discuss the subject of empathy can be confusing. Empathy is a form of emotional connection that is accessible to almost everyone on the planet, but an empath is more than simply a person who experiences empathetic feelings. An individual with healthy empathetic sensibilities can use their empathy as a tool when circumstances call for it, but an empath often doesn't have the option of putting that tool away or choosing when, where, and how to apply it. Some empaths see their heightened sensitivity as a gift, but many others find it frustrating and difficult to manage.

To understand how heightened empathy can be challenging, we'll first need to understand empathy as a necessary element in human development, as well as how higher, lower or average degrees of empathic sensitivity affect interpersonal dynamics.

What is Empathy?

Empathy. It's something all humans are capable of feeling and expressing, to some degree or other, and yet in these modern times, there never seems to be quite enough of it to go around.

When most of us talk about empathy, we think of it as the virtue that must be coupled with any other positive character trait for it to be considered truly good. A generous or charitable nature, without empathy, can look at lots like condescension or a controlling attitude. Optimism and positivity, without empathy, can seem insensitive or even mean-spirited to those who are suffering. Kindness and love, without empathy, can become dangerous infatuation, which might feel truly threatening to those on the receiving end of these emotions. Empathy is the root of all nuances in our day-to-day interactions. Without it, the concept of respect would be impossible to describe or display; there would be no such thing as contagious or infectious laughter. There would be no joy (or anxiety) to be found in any traditional exchange of gifts; we would never be moved to tears by any film or work of art, and it's entirely possible that there would be no such thing as pornography.

All of these facets of human society are heavily reliant on

empathy--not sympathy, for which empathy is commonly mistaken. Sympathy is the mental exercise of imagining how you might feel if you stood in another person's shoes; this is the attitude which allows us to walk past a homeless person in the wintertime, and silently acknowledge that they might be cold, hungry, exhausted, or sad. Sympathy propels us to say, either aloud or in our heads: "I feel bad for that person," or "that must be a really difficult life."

Empathy takes this idea a step further. It is not just a mental exercise. When we share empathy with a homeless person in wintertime, we don't only theoretically put ourselves in their position--we allow our emotional or physical states to be deeply affected by their circumstances. We may feel cold and shivery ourselves, or become saddened, carrying a sudden feeling of hopelessness or isolation; furthermore, we might have trouble letting go of those feelings for a long while after we leave that environment, for hours, days, or even weeks.

Sympathy is not a bad thing by any means; it will frequently inspire a passing pedestrian to search their pockets for spare change and cash to offer a person in need. But someone who feels empathy for the homeless, rather than sympathy, might be more likely to stop even if they have no money to give. Empathy might allow you to realize that money isn't the only thing of value that you could offer them; instead, you might note that they are largely ignored, that they must feel somewhat invisible, and so you would make a point to smile and greet them, whether or not you have any change to spare. In simpler terms, sympathy is what allows us to acknowledge the feelings of other people, while empathy is what allows us to share their emotional experiences as if they were our own.

Empathy and sympathy are both fluids--these are not fixed traits, but rather skills that can be honed and strengthened, or grow weak from misuse over time. You may go through periods of your life wherein you find it easy to walk past a person in need without a second thought, and yet feel that it's impossible to ignore them at other times. But there is a certain degree of empathic ability that is currently considered standard or average for most humans--we tend to feel stronger empathy in childhood. As adults, we learn to regulate our emotional responses and distinguish them from other people's, deciding when and where it's most appropriate to display empathy, or to keep our feelings to ourselves.

When empathy is present to a useful degree, it is not typically measured, since it is displayed in varied forms from one person to another, and we still do not have commonly agreed upon metrics by which to evaluate it. But we rely on the standard degree of empathy for so many of our interpersonal connections, that most of us tend only to notice when it is missing from an interaction, rather than when it is present, like oxygen. It feels natural to most of us to rearrange our facial muscles and display concern when we face someone who is crying or obviously in distress; therefore, if we note someone is smiling or laughing in response to another person's misery, we can immediately sense that something is "off."

Within the past few decades, the fields of psychology, neuroscience, and many others have made enormous strides in research towards understanding the minds of those who do not display the "normal" amount of empathy. There are some conditions, such as autism or Asperger's syndrome, wherein a person seems able to detect the emotional energies of those around them, but lacks the necessary cognitive tools to interpret them or determine an appropriate reaction. These people often feel attacked or overwhelmed when the emotions of others resonate within them, which is a form of empathic sensitivity, but they often react by shutting down or self-isolating rather than trying to find a way to harmonious coexistence. It is not a struggle for these people to put their own needs first in interpersonal connections, even if it is at the expense of other people's feelings, but this isn't a malicious sentiment; it is primarily a self-preservation instinct in hyper-drive.

Alternatively, there are empathy-deficient personality disorders, such as narcissism, sociopathy, and psychopathy, wherein a person is capable of recognizing the emotions of others, but feels personally detached from them. That is why we often describe psychopathic criminals as "cold" or "calculating." It is unsettling to imagine that a person could decide to take action, knowing that their behavior will cause pain or suffering in others and that they might remain unbothered by that factor or derive pleasure from it--but that is the thought process of an empathy-disordered individual. The feelings of others are considered unimportant because they do not impact their emotional sensations.

The general population holds a lot of misconceptions about people with these personality disorders, which are most evident within the criminal justice system. Many of us convince ourselves, for instance, that these people commit crimes of passion, temporarily losing their sense of right and wrong in the blinding heat of rage, or that they are so mentally skewed as to be incapable of understanding how much pain and suffering they are causing. Unfortunately, neither of these possibilities proves true for these individuals. They do understand the impact of their actions and are capable of determining right from wrong, yet they choose to ignore these factors, hurting other people to serve strategic needs or for the sake of personal gain. People with these personality disorders generally display impressive skill with cognitive empathy, which you might think of as theoretical empathy; this allows them to theorize or predict the emotional reactions of others and makes them masterful manipulators.

When discussing those who struggle to display or feel empathy, it's important to remember that empathic abilities are fluid, not fixed in stone; anyone willing to put in the effort can improve their empathic capabilities, even those who have been diagnosed with an empathy deficient condition or disorder. Physical empathy is often accessible to those who do not display emotional empathy, which may be a function of evolutionary development. Humans can better protect their physical bodies by recognizing physical pain in others and are biologically driven to mimic pleasurable behaviors (whether that means eating good food or enjoying sexual stimulation) by watching others and empathizing with their enjoyment of such activities. Since this form of empathy is often observable in scans of empathy-disordered brains, we must embrace the notion that empathy exists as a complex and fluid and scale; it is not like a light switch that is either flipped on or off.

If everyone is capable of empathy, then how is an Empath different from anyone else?

The words "empath" and "empathy" both stem from the Ancient Greek term "Empatheia," which is a hybrid of the words "en" meaning "in" or "at" and "pathos" which means "passion" or "feeling", but can also be interpreted to mean "suffering." It is etymological root is perfectly illustrative of empathy as a double-edged sword. Humans crave deep interpersonal connection and often find joy in shared passions, but when we open ourselves up to the blessings of those around us, we also open ourselves up to their sorrows, fears, and furies.

This struggle, ultimately, is where we can draw a line between average empathetic instinct, and true empathic sensitivity. Most people can choose to detach or distance themselves from empathic sensations if they become overwhelming, distracting, or unpleasant, but the empath cannot help but tune into the emotional energies surrounding them--even if such a connection is detrimental to their well-being. Empaths are equally likely to share in another person's joy or suffering, which means many of them are forced to carry more than their fair share of emotional (or physical) pain through life.

Often, people mistake the concept of empathic power for the rare supernatural gifts of clairvoyance, telepathy, or predictive ability. But empaths may not have any sense of seeing the future before it plays out. They very rarely claim to receive messages from deceased spirits or to be able to channel precise, detailed notes to other living beings without verbal contact. Many empaths struggle with metaphysical or spiritual concepts and do not personally believe in any supernatural power. They can be clumsy without much skill for proprioception; they might have a poor sense of direction, and frequently get lost; they can appear flighty and easily confused; they might strike you as spaced out, flaky, or oblivious to their surroundings; and they may display poor social skills in certain situations.

A person who claims to be an empath isn't necessarily saying they can read minds or predict the future; most empaths are merely tuned in to specific energetic frequencies which most people are not sensitive to, and this sensitivity is usually involuntary. Untrained or unawakened empaths especially do not get to choose whether or not external energies impact them. Sometimes, empaths are so sharply attuned to these frequencies that they have trouble reading other surface-level indicators of energetic vibration. For example, an emotional empath may be highly sensitive to the emotional sensations of others around them, and particularly apt at detecting these energies through audio sensory perception--so much so, that visual cues might serve to confuse or distort the messages they receive sonically. This type of empath might need to keep their eyes closed to strengthen their sonic sensitivity and avoid confusion, as well as exhaustion from cognitive dissonance. Alternatively, another empath may rely on visual clues, or sense energetic frequencies physically through touch, and find any auditory stimulus distracting or overwhelming. Furthermore, there are some empath types whose empathy doesn't serve them in interpersonal connection at all, yet they can pick up on the energetic vibrations of animals, plants, inanimate objects or places.

Where does empathic power come from?

The question of where empathic powers come from, or how people come to possess them, is one that science still does not have a solid answer. But there are a few theories. There is indeed plenty of evidence to suggest that a "normal" degree of empathy is accessible to most of us in early development. Newborn infants in neonatal units display an inability to distinguish personal feelings from those around them; if one infant begins to cry, usually most others will follow suit very quickly, as they are not yet aware that this pain or anxiety isn't theirs to own. Most infants who receive a healthy amount of care and attention will continue mimicry and emotional enmeshment throughout the first few years of life--this is how children can learn speech and movement. Some children, raised in especially tight-knit families or communities, may struggle at first to understand the function of pronouns that distinguish between the individual self and the group, posing questions like, "Mama, why are we sad today?" when they observe this emotion in another person.

Those who believe in the supernatural possibilities of empathic power also tend to think that certain individuals are fated to receive these gifts and that empaths feel as they do to serve some higher purpose as determined by cosmic or holy design. This belief often coincides with the notion that empaths are born unique, and not shaped by their surroundings; while the level of power they possess or how they channel energy may fluctuate throughout their lives, their heightened sensitivity is considered an innate trait.

Conversely, there are those who believe empathic abilities come from the environment or circumstances in which a person is raised, as a function of nurture rather than nature. Many psychologists note that children raised in volatile, neglectful, or dangerous households learn early on to detect subtle changes in their parents' behaviors as a necessary coping skill and defense mechanism, allowing them to predict, avoid, or even prevent traumatic episodes.

Parents may not necessarily be evil or malicious in raising a child who develops extreme empathic sensitivity. Some theories posit that the only environmental factor needed to trigger such a development is an older authoritative figure in the child's life which requires the child to empathize with them frequently. For example, a parent who is grieving the loss of a loved one might, without ever intending to, compel their child to empathize with a level of emotional pain which they haven't yet been prepared for, and can hardly even comprehend at such a young age. A child who is put in this position frequently enough may never learn to distinguish their own emotions from those of others, and might even struggle to feel that they are real, substantial, or whole without the influence of another dominant personality. They become hyper-focused on caring for the parental figure in their life, and never learn how to receive care without guilt, shame or anxiety, as most children do.

Once a child develops this ability, it is only natural for them to continue using it outside the home, amongst friends, colleagues, lovers, and even strangers. There are also those who note this same skill of hyper-sensitivity emerging for the first time in full-grown adults when they are romantically involved (or otherwise firmly bonded) with an abusive personality type, such as a narcissist.

It is worth noting that many empaths first become aware of their heightened sensitivity during relationships with those who are empathy deficient. Furthermore, whether they are aware of their abilities or not, empaths are so frequently involved with narcissists, sociopaths and psychopaths, that many wonders if empathic power functions as a sort of invisible beacon to those who have these personality disorders. The theory that empaths and empathy deficient types are drawn to each other like magnets begs the question- which typically comes first? The empathic power or the abusive environment in which it becomes a necessary skill for survival? While it makes sense that empathic abilities develop as a response to abuse and trauma, it is also certainly possible that abuse and trauma would always exist anyways, and empaths are merely drawn to these environments more than most people. An unfortunate reality of life for the empath who has not yet fully awakened to their power is that they will often feel compassion for those whom everyone else has abandoned, failing to see that these souls have been left alone for a good reason and are not worthy of the empath's care or attention. It could indicate that abusive circumstances and relationships are like traps which empaths are particularly vulnerable to falling into, rather than the cause or catalyst for heightened sensitivity.

Thus far, science has not been able to provide proof one way or the other, but some recent findings may allow for both possibilities to coexist. The study of epigenetics concerns how our genetic material is impacted by our experiences and surroundings, meaning that we pass on more to our children through our DNA than merely a blueprint for the body. With the discovery of epigenetics, we are now able to theorize that trauma can have an intergenerational ripple effect, leaving a lasting mark on the descendants of victims, whether those descendants are fully aware of the trauma or not. That would allow a soul to be born with empathic abilities which are at once innate and a developed response to abuse.

There are many possible sources of empathic ability, and new information is continually surfacing to expand our understanding of it. Likewise, the scientific field has yet to firmly define the cause of empathy-deficient personality disorders, nor that of conditions like autism and Asperger's syndrome. Some believe these emotional states or conditions feed into one another, like two species sharing a symbiotic relationship, or an actual embodiment of yin and yang energies. Others still believe there are purely biological explanations for conditions that fall on both ends of the empathy scale. Then, of course, there are those who see the empathy scale as a circle rather than a line, believing that a person with an overabundance of new empathic ability can evolve into a narcissist or vice versa.

Whatever you believe, one thing is clear. Empathic ability must be understood, trained, and balanced to be part of a healthy, happy lifestyle. In the next chapter, you can evaluate the strength of your empathic sensitivity and determine how much energy to channel into further education, training, and healing.

2

Are you an Empath? Self-assessment Test

If the descriptions of empathic ability in the last chapter struck a familiar chord, you might be wondering now if you are empath yourself. It's entirely possible that you are, especially if you felt compelled to purchase this book; those with personality types that are deficient in empathy are generally unbothered by the deficiency, and thus aren't curious to learn more about the empathic qualities they lack. Additionally, the average person is capable of empathizing under circumstances wherein their empathy can be beneficial to them, but most can turn this impulse off, if and when such a connection becomes challenging, unpleasant, or debilitating. For those who can use empathy like a muscle, putting it to work when necessary and leaving it to rest when it is not useful, empathy rarely presents a problem, and thus, they may not feel any impetus to understand the concept more deeply.

If you have found your way to this survival guide, chances are you have not been quite so lucky. Perhaps you've seen yourself struggling to shake off negative thoughts or feelings, even while your rational brain believes you should be over them by now. Maybe you've had difficulty lately in recognizing the boundaries between your own emotions and those of your friends, family, or colleagues. You might be plagued with feelings of confusion, or a sense of being frequently overwhelmed by phantom stressors. These are all signs that your empathic abilities are stronger than those of the average individual, and that you may need to develop strategies to protect your emotional balance and stay grounded in the self.

The question of whether or not you have empathy is an easy one to answer. Have you felt compelled to smile witnessing a stranger receive a gift? Or felt moved to tears over someone else's sorrow? Have you ever felt amused by the sight of another person laughing, even if you didn't understand what they found so funny? Have you felt woozy or nauseous at the sight of someone else's injury? Or, have you found yourself mirroring a friend's wide-mouthed yawns, even if you didn't feel the least bit tired? These are all examples of common empathetic connections; almost everyone is familiar with one or more of these experiences, the notable exception being those with empathy deficient personality disorders like psychopathy, sociopathy, and narcissism.

So where can we draw the line between average, run-of-the-mill empathy, and the type of empathic power that needs to be proactively managed? One easy answer is to apply the same standards that we use to identify problematic addictions. For instance, eating is something everyone has to do, but members of organizations like Overeaters Anonymous identify the practice as an addiction when it becomes more than merely a question of necessity, convenience, or pleasure. When a person's eating habits become compulsive or irrational and leave them struggling to manage other areas of life, food stops being a form of fuel or a biological imperative. Instead, it becomes a force exerting power over their emotional, mental, and physical capacities. Just as a food addict might feel unable to resist another bite, even if their stomach is already in pain from overeating, an empath may be unable to resist emotional involvement with others, maybe allowing (or inviting) a friend to sob on their shoulder over a recent job loss even though the empath is already overwhelmed with personal grief.

Empathy in itself is not a problematic entity; the issue is that empaths tend to feel it too intensely, too often, and sometimes allow it to control their lives. Since it is an internal thought process rather than an external substance or activity, this is an especially tricky addiction to manage; and ultimately, you don't stand a chance at maintaining your empathic abilities until you are ready to acknowledge their existence, recognize their impact on every aspect of your life, and mentally prepare yourself to embrace their power.

Self-assessment Test

Read the statements below to yourself, and keep a careful note of how many of them you agree with. Use a piece of paper and pen to tally the number of times you identify with the statements--this number will be your empathic score. If you agree strongly and frequently with a statement, mark down 2 points. If you agree somewhat, occasionally, or under specific circumstances, mark down 1 point for yourself. If you do not identify or agree with a statement at all, mark down 0 points.

Try to be as honest with yourself as possible. Answer with your gut, and don't overthink your responses. Also, remember that this self-assessment is designed to evaluate your current empathic abilities, which are fluid and in constant fluctuation. If you find you are torn on any statements, perhaps because you once identified strongly with them but now you no longer do, or vice versa, choose whatever answer resonates most powerfully with your present-day self.

If this produces results that you find disappointing, don't let yourself get discouraged. Remember that empathic abilities can always grow, transform and evolve, especially if you are actively pursuing that growth. A low score today does not necessarily mean you possess an empathy-deficient personality disorder, nor is it a permanent result--it may just be an indication that your current surroundings, coping mechanisms, relationships or habits are stifling your empathic capabilities, and a change may be necessary before you can begin to sharpen your skills. Likewise, a high score is not something to simply congratulate yourself for and then forget. Empathic abilities, like muscles, need to be trained, fueled, and adequately cared for to maintain their strength; if you do not use them, you are likely to lose them.

It might be best to take this quiz when you are alone, calm, and able to focus, attending to no one else's needs but your own. If you are indeed an empath, your answers may be impacted by the feelings, judgments, or values of others around you, which can ultimately skew your scoring results.

1. I feel emotions more deeply than most.
2. I have been called "very sensitive," or perhaps even "too sensitive," by others.
3. I can become overwhelmed or uncomfortable in large crowds.
4. I sometimes feel the need for complete, uninterrupted solitude (maybe with quiet and or darkness, but not sleep) to gather my thoughts or "recharge" my energy.
5. I can tell when people are lying or trying to mask

their feelings, even if no one else around seems to see it.
6. I am very conscious of how my actions will affect those around me.
7. I find the emotional reactions of other people-- laughing, crying, scowling in anger-- be genuinely contagious, regardless of the emotional state I bring to the interaction; even if I am over-the-moon with personal joy, I can be quickly moved to tears by someone else's sorrow.
8. I am deeply bothered by situations of injustice, and often can't help but try to find a solution or remedy, even if it's none of my business or beyond my reach to do so.
9. I am drawn to animals, and I am more comfortable with them than in the company of some humans.
10. I am often told that I am a great listener.
11. I tend to take care of others before I address my own needs.
12. My emotional reactions seem to last longer than they do for other people--it might take me days or weeks to get over something that other people move on from in a matter of hours.
13. In a phone call (or another form of communication where I can't see someone's face) I can read someone's emotional state just from the sound of their voice, and usually gather this from only one or two words of greeting.

Empath

14. There are certain forms of graphic media that I just can't stomach--violence, for instance, or humiliation-based comedy is almost painful for me to watch, and I find it hard to shake the feeling off even after it's over.
15. People often open up to me, even those I don't know very well, sharing secrets, confessions, or other pieces of intimate knowledge.
16. I often find myself getting emotionally involved in other people's problems or successes; I might be deeply distraught over a friend's break-up or thrilled when a colleague receives a well-deserved promotion.
17. I frequently catch myself mirroring the body language of others, or mimicking accents and patterns of speech, during conversations.
18. I am more sensitive than most to temperature, and usually, feel chilly in places where others are perfectly comfortable.
19. I can't help reading between the lines or hearing the subtext of a conversation just as loudly as what is articulated verbally.
20. My emotions tend to resonate throughout my entire body; I have a hard time compartmentalizing or ignoring them.
21. I sometimes experience synesthesia, where two or more of my sensory perceptions are intertwined (a sensation of feeling color, perhaps, or seeing

sounds, associating numerical values with musical notes, or feeling that certain days or months are linked to locations or emotional states, etcetera.)
22. I can be easily distracted by an external stimulus.
23. Anything that feels inauthentic--a book or movie, a business, or even someone's personality--is a huge turnoff for me, and I cannot stand to be around such things for more than a few minutes without experiencing pain or discomfort.
24. I do not mind being alone if I can determine how I send the time; I might prefer to stay home on Saturday night to read or paint or cook, rather than attend a party.
25. I am susceptible to bright lights, odors, and sounds, sometimes profoundly bothered by them while others can easily ignore them.
26. When conflict arises between people I know but does not involve me, I still feel hurt, angry, confused or sad, and I am preoccupied until I've taken action to encourage peacemaking.
27. Miscommunication is profoundly frustrating for me to experience or witness, even between strangers.
28. I can sometimes experience two or more contrasting emotions simultaneously; I might be full of joy and fear and sadness, feeling each emotion equally and all at once.
29. I feel deeply connected to underdogs, both in entertainment media and in real life. I can be

Empath

protective of friends and total strangers alike-- anyone who seems especially vulnerable to victimization.

30. I have trouble accepting absolutes, believing that anyone is purely good or evil, that anything is decisively the best or the worst of its kind; I think the truth is always complex, multifaceted, and fluid, because it is largely a matter of perspective.
31. It is sometimes challenging for me to stay present at the moment; my mind is often stuck in the past or fixed in the future.
32. I react to most stimuli quickly and viscerally; I am not the type to sit back and wait to see how things play out before I decide how to feel about the situation.
33. Watching group interactions can be fascinating to me; I sometimes feel as if I can see or sense a complex web of emotions tying every member of the group together, like a game of cat's cradle, influencing their movements, behaviors, and attitudes.
34. The planned trajectories of my days can be thrown off course by fairly small triggers. Something as small as a sharp exchange, a missed green light, a good sign or bad omen, even a momentary sense of deja vu, might cast a ripple effect on my itinerary for the rest of the day or even week.
35. Music, movies, books, dance, and other art forms

often give me a sense of being entirely transported to a different time, place, and reality; or, they might trigger an out-of-body experience for me. They can deliver a feeling of transcendence, even if I have no reason to identify with them.

36. I have an eye for small details that others frequently overlook.
37. When I connect with someone I like, we often form an extraordinarily deep bond, and we do so very quickly.
38. Conversely, I often meet people and immediately get bad feelings about them without being able to explain why. That may even be the case if the person in question displays kindness towards me at a surface level, which makes me even more uncomfortable.
39. I don't usually dominate conversations, or feel comfortable talking about myself for long periods. I tend to listen or ask questions to encourage input from everyone involved.
40. I have a talent for bringing shy children, adults, or animals, out of their shells.
41. If I am immersed in a creative pursuit or interest (reading, research, sculpture, dance, whatever sparks your passion) I can get lost in it for hours or even days. I might forget to eat or take care of other necessities because of it.
42. I have vivid, elaborate dreams, frequent episodes of

deja vu, or surreal, out-of-body sensations. (Score 1 if you experience one or two regularly; score two if you experience all three once in a while, or any of the above with high frequency.)

43. I am very particular about what I eat. I'm sensitive to flavors, textures, temperatures, and whether or not the food in question has been ethically sourced. These things impact my enjoyment of the eating experience, as well as the way my body feels afterwards throughout the entire digestive process.

44. I have a rich, complex, detailed inner world. Sometimes, it seems impossible to convey what I carry inside of me to the outside world or to adequately express my thoughts and beliefs. I often experience emotions or sensations, and then realize that there is no word in existence to describe what I'm feeling.

45. I tend to notice that which fades into the background for others; for instance, at a play or dance performance, I might look past the lead and become fixated on watching a particular chorus member, or shadows of stage-hands in the wings. I can easily see past distraction tactics or showy displays.

46. Organization and efficiency are vital to me and come naturally. I can quickly pinpoint flaws in organizational systems by imagining myself in the shoes of all the people who use them.

47. I have a hard time understanding how some people distance themselves from intense emotions. If I feel bliss, grief, rage, shame, or love, I feel it thoroughly, and these emotions sometimes consume me.
48. I get stomach aches, indigestion, headaches, or other physical symptoms in concert with emotions like anxiety or melancholy. These symptoms are sometimes triggered when I know people around me are struggling with these emotions, while I am otherwise content.
49. Nuance stands out to me; it can either be delightful or ruin my enjoyment of an otherwise pleasant experience.
50. I find it hard to say "no" to anything people ask of me, even if compliance will be detrimental to my well-being.
51. I often feel completely overwhelmed or engulfed by my concerns or anxieties, only to realize later that my worries were irrational, or that I made a mountain out of a molehill.
52. I may be a neat freak, or if I am not, I am very particular about the way I keep my living space and have a system for everything. If something in my space has been moved or tampered with, I can immediately sense that something is off.
53. I don't usually feel like I fit in with those around me, even people who love and appreciate me.
54. When I am stressed, sad, or otherwise unhappy, I

tend to turn to indulgences or vices for comfort--sexual stimulation, alcohol or drug use, overeating, gambling, etc.
55. I feel most energized by nature and solitude.
56. Conversations with some people exhaust me as much as an intense physical workout; I need to rest and recover afterwards before I can engage with anyone else.
57. When I answer the phone or run into an old friend in public, I often find myself saying: "That's so funny; I was just thinking, talking, and dreaming about you!"
58. Clothing and accessories aren't just adornment--for me; they're more like armor. I may have certain tender areas like my abdomen, chest or throat that I prefer to keep densely covered with thick, plush fabrics, and shielded behind large belts, chunky jewelry, etc.
59. I don't aim to cut people off or interject rudely, but when someone is struggling to find the right words to finish a sentence, I'm usually able to fill in the blanks for them, and they're most often grateful for the words I offer, saying: "Yes, that's exactly the term I was looking for!"
60. I have lots of allergies and sensitivities related to my skin and or digestive system.

Your score

Tally up all your zeroes, ones and twos to find your current position on the empathy quotient scale. Remember not to let these numbers discourage you, or give you too big of a head--empathy is fluid, and there is always room for growth!

0-20 - Little to no empathic connection

If fewer than twenty of these questions resonated with you, don't interpret that to mean you are incapable of empathy. This score might indicate an empathy deficient condition or disorder, but it also could come from an individual with average, or even heightened, empathic abilities who have learned to close themselves off temporarily. People sometimes reject or turn away from empathic sensitivity as a response to being hurt, having their ego severely bruised, experiencing trauma or grief, as a reaction to long periods of solitude, or a lack of privacy and personal space. Whatever the reason for your score, try to view this number as a jumping off point to start building your empathic energy. Try this test again in a few months, and you may be pleasantly surprised by your growth.

20-40 - Average empathic sensitivity

You are sensitive to the world around you, but selectively. You have a healthy sense of self, you know what you like, and you understand your value system. You recognize the boundary between your own emotions and other people's feelings but can still empathize fully in appropriate situations.

At this position on the empathy quotient scale, your boundaries need to be strong. If you surround yourself with people who display low empathetic sensitivity levels, you may find your score gradually decreases under their influence.

40-80 - Heightened empathic ability

Your empathic capability is above average, but perhaps not so strong that you have been forced to reckon with it entirely. You've found it helpful in some ways, but profoundly confusing and frustrating at times, too. That can be a turbulent awakening experience, as empathetic sensations come to you seemingly from out of nowhere, unpredictably and often at extremely inconvenient times. If your sensitivity is awakened but not trained, you are vulnerable to the whims of the world, like a rowboat in the sea without a paddle. You'll first want to enhance your empathic sensitivity and understanding, and then determine the specifics of your empathic type, before ultimately learning how to balance and ground your energy.

80-120 - Advanced empathic power

This score could alternatively be called "severe empathic sensitivity," depending on how well you've managed your abilities thus far. You feel a great deal more empathy than most, which leaves you quite vulnerable to toxic energy, emotional contagion, and depletion. With education, training and spiritual guidance, you'll be able to manage your power and maintain your energy levels, but it will take plenty of focus, determination, and patience to reach a point of emotional stability. With this degree of power, your reach may very well exceed your grasp, so it's important to seek out experienced mentors, metaphysical healers, and spiritual teachers to help guide you to a place of deeper understanding.

3

Common Traits of the Empath

An empath will usually know if they like someone or not very quickly after meeting them. When empaths meet someone showy, inauthentic or cynical, they may immediately get an indescribable "bad feeling" combined with the impulse to get as far away from the person as they possibly can. Alternatively, they may decide upon a first meeting that a person seems honest or kind-hearted, even though it's impossible to discern such knowledge from one interaction alone. Empaths often cross paths with people and sense their need for emotional or physical healing right away, providing a listening ear, shoulder to cry on, or maybe even a healing touch if it's accessible to them.

Their sharp emotional perceptions shape them into strange, atypical social animals. They feel deep compassion for underdogs and detest blatant displays of narcissism, so they tend to attract social outcasts like moths to a flame. Empaths may have a vast and diverse array of friends, but they may also appear to have more enemies than the average person, as they are susceptible, easily hurt, and often unwilling to feign social niceties. Oddly enough, many empaths report having a large number of friends, and yet only knowing one or two people that they feel genuinely close.

Sometimes, though, the empath can get lucky and cross paths with someone that they click with right away--someone who seems to "just get it" without having any deep knowledge about the empath's background or personal circumstances. This person doesn't just win the empath over with their charisma or kindness--instead, they seem to vibrate at the same energetic frequency. Together as fast friends, they might discover all kinds of bizarre little coincidences--not just common likes and dislikes, but also similar allergies and ailments, everyday habits, unusual preferences and tastes, family and social backgrounds, and on and on.

Perhaps without even knowing it, two empaths have found one another.

Hopefully, you'll be lucky enough to experience this fantastic connection many times throughout your life. When you are lucky, do your best to nurture and protect your friendships with other empaths, even if they have not yet fully awakened to their emotional body or energetic identity. Empaths, specially empowered ones, can recharge each other's energy stores in ways that most other people can't. Forming a network of fellow empaths will serve to make everyone involved stronger and happier; you will heal each other, lift each other, support each other, and stabilize each other.

There are many different types of empaths, which we'll discuss in detail in the next chapter. If you had a high empathic score in the self-assessment test from the previous chapter, it would benefit you to befriend any empath you encounter, whether you sense energies through the same medium or not.

It just so happens that your author identifies as an empath, and has spent a great deal of time learning how to recognize and attract kindred spirits. Here are some traits that I've found to be overwhelmingly common amongst empaths of all types. This list should help you to spot your fellow empaths out in the wild, and maybe find a deeper understanding of yourself in the process.

- **We are expressive** - Empaths may not speak loudly or often, but when we do speak up, what we have to say is rarely boring. We may be wordsmiths or casual poets. We might be the type to gesticulate wildly or act stories out while we tell them. Stoicism usually only shows up in empaths who are uncomfortable or distracted.
- **We are introverts** - This trait will be discussed at great length in the following chapters, because it may be a direct result of empathic ability. Empaths

often feel exhausted by the emotions of others and need regular time alone to recharge. This trait should not be confused for social anxiety or shyness. We can still be outgoing; we can still enjoy the occasional party or a night on the town, and we still cherish time spent with our loved ones. We simply find that being around others can drain us rather than energize us, and we need periodic solitude to recuperate.

- **We are people pleasers** - We can sense what people want from us, and furthermore, we can feel the disappointment we cause in others when we refuse whatever is asked of us. It can be easier to say yes to everything at first simply, but this is a tough practice to sustain. We are prone to burning ourselves out while trying to make everyone else happy, forgetting to take care of our own needs.

- **We are very particular** - Empaths notice all the minor details so that we can develop extremely specific tastes. It can apply to the way we like to consume our food and beverages, the conditions we need to sleep comfortably, the way we like our living spaces arranged, the fabrics we wear, and more. It may seem over-the-top if we are picky about the percentage of milk fat in a cup of coffee, but some of us really can taste the difference between 1% and 2% milk, and it doesn't seem minor to us.

- **We seem unfocused** - Empaths are fickle creatures full of contradictions. Many of us could be seen as neat freaks based on the way we manage our living or workspaces. At the same time, outside of those limited environments, we can appear wildly disorganized, flaky and forgetful. It is especially true for those of us who haven't yet learned to maintain our boundaries or protect our energetic fields. We are quite vulnerable to distraction.
- **We are human mirrors** - Sometimes, empaths can put people off through mimicry. We usually don't mean anything by it, though; our impulse to mirror people in conversation is automatic, and often, we don't even realize we are doing it. We yawn when we see other people yawn; we adopt their hand gestures, postures, and patterns of speech; we might even seem to be mocking foreign accents, though again, we usually don't intend any harm or offense. When we try to suppress these impulses, it can make us look twitchy or nervous.
- **If it's fake, we want nothing to do with it** - Authenticity is deeply valuable to empaths, so anything that feels inauthentic can be uncomfortable or even painful for us to tolerate. It can apply to entertainment media, businesses, or people around us. It also makes it difficult for us to pretend we are happy when we aren't, or mask any

emotion for the sake of other people's comfort. We are generally kind-hearted, but we can also be brutally honest at times because lying is physically unpleasant for us. We might become especially tactless when we are exhausted.

- **We cry a lot** - Whether they're tears of joy, sorrow, or confusion, we get choked up very quickly. Empaths are often the type to cry over television commercials or social media posts. Attending the weddings or funerals of people we don't know, we will still end up sobbing for hours. Some of us even have automatic tearing reflexes to certain sounds, flavors, sensations or conceptual ideas.

- **We can't stop our emotions from manifesting in our bodies** - Empaths often appear volatile or erratic to those who don't understand us, because we wear our feelings so plainly on our sleeves. We are often unable to suppress smiles or laughter, even if the circumstances call for us to stay straight-faced. If we are involved in, or even just near a conflict, we may get hot red cheeks and elevated heartbeat, white knuckles and popping veins in our temples. If we watch someone endure an embarrassment or humiliation, we might become nauseated, or suddenly feel unable to stand upright. When an empath tells someone, "I feel your pain," we rarely mean this figuratively.

- **We are creative** - Empaths are deeply observant, and many of us struggle to find appropriate audiences to share our feelings. With such a rich, complex inner world of unexpressed thought to draw from, we are often visionary creatives, seeking to translate our feelings into a medium that can move others as powerfully as the sentiments of others move us. We are painters, singers, dancers, actors, and sculptors; many of us have talents for fictional world-building, film direction or production, architecture and city planning, fashion design, orchestral composition, and other creative projects of enormous scale. We often have a peculiar knack for seeing the big picture and focusing on small details simultaneously.

- **We are misunderstood** - Creative as we may be; mundane verbal expression is not typically the empath's strong point. We are usually uncomfortable talking about ourselves or peacocking, so sometimes, creative expression is the only form of expression we project outward into the world. To make matters even more confusing, we tend to mimic the behaviors of those we spend time with and have weak emotional boundaries. It makes it even harder for others to read us or figure us out. To the casual observer, we can appear moody or melodramatic; or, if we have learned to temper our emotional displays in social situations, we might seem aloof and detached. These impressions will no doubt fade away for those who get to know us; they'll discover that in truth, empaths usually make excellent, stable, loving, trustworthy friends.

- **We are daydreamers** - Since we are misunderstood, many of us are used to keeping our thoughts and revelations to ourselves. We can often get lost for long periods in our thoughts, either planning some new creative endeavor, ruminating on past experiences, or just trying to sort out the root of a current emotion.

- **We tend to run cold** - This is intended to be read literally, not figuratively (though you may find an empath's disposition quite chilly at times, too). We are sensitive to climate and temperature changes of all kinds, no matter how minor, and generally, we tend to feel cold where others are perfectly comfortable. We like to be cozy, and usually prefer modest, warm clothing. We need full coverage from our bedspreads to sleep, even in the heat of summer.

- **We are peacemakers** - Empaths can see both sides of most arguments, and they can feel the tension and anger on both sides, too. We desperately wish that those in conflict could see what we see. A peaceful resolution helps us all to feel better in the end, but the journey is getting there can be draining for the empath.

- **We can manage a crisis like it's our job** - When chaos erupts, or an emergency arises, empaths often surprise everyone (including themselves) by stepping up and displaying sudden confidence, taking charge of the situation and triaging priorities. Perhaps this is because we can sense the conflict and tension in a room so powerfully that we feel the need to remedy it as a form of self-preservation. We are usually able to help hysterical people calm down quickly, and know how to make an injured person as comfortable as possible. We can read a room in pandemonium, analyzing and evaluating the varying degrees of urgency required to fix each problem in turn.

- **At the same time, we can be easily overwhelmed** - Outside of an emergency or crisis, empaths might have a very tough time adjusting to changing plans, going with the flow, handling unexpected events, or simply existing within a group where each person wants something different. We tend to envision or feel the future ripple effects of any choice, so it's hard for us to make decisions lightly. We also see the potential for small problems to spiral into larger ones, so we can

easily overreact to minor issues.
- **We are better at solving other people's problems than our own** - The empath can detect the unspoken and unseen for others, but often we have a blind spot in ourselves. I know one empath who visits the houses of friends or strangers to help them find things they've lost in their clutter; if the item is accurately described to her, she can usually locate it within a minute, even if it's hidden someplace genuinely unpredictable. In her own home, however, she might spend a full hour searching for something right in front of her nose. That is a common challenge for empaths, especially in our emotional lives, which is why we might detest narcissistic personality traits, and still somehow end up married to a malignant narcissist.
- **We feel emotional pain and suffering intensely** - This is true even if the pain shouldn't be ours to bear. It means some of us can't be around our friends for extended visits when they are in the throes of emotional anguish. It also implies some of us cannot bear to watch violent movies or even the news.
- **We hurt a lot** - Many of us suffer from chronic aches, pains, illnesses and injuries that we can't seem to explain. These pains may reflect specific injuries to other people's bodies, or they may be a sort of general accumulation of unpleasant

physical and emotional sensations picked up from our surroundings. For this reason, many of us also find we are incapable of causing pain to anyone around us, even in the name of self-defense. We are driven to heal, not hurt. Ironically, our healing nature seems to draw suffering people towards us, so our loving relationships may bring us just as much pain as joy.

- **We are selfless to a fault** - Empowered empaths may have learned to temper this impulse in the name of balance, but generally speaking, we are people who give too much to others, and only realize later that we haven't saved anything for ourselves. We often put everyone else's needs before our own, sometimes to the degree that seems absurd to others. An easy illustration is holding doors in public places; empaths are the types of people who often get stuck holding a door open at a busy train station, letting six, eight, ten people pass through before realizing they'll miss their train if they don't butt into the line soon. It is challenging for us to remember that we cannot serve anyone water from an empty well.

- **We see connections and coincidences everywhere** - We are very sensitive to minor details, so we tend to note synchronicities that most people overlook. These connections are everywhere, and they are confusing to navigate when nobody else seems to see them. We might sound a bit like conspiracy theorists, but usually, we're just trying to make sense of a collection of information we've drawn from varied perspectives.

- **We have addictive personalities** - This doesn't necessarily have to apply to vices or risky behaviors, but when empaths get into something, we tend to go all the way down the rabbit hole with it. That might be because little rushes of dopamine or adrenaline can help us to temporarily block out the energy pollution we pick up just by being around other people, and that sense of relief is ultimately more addictive for us than whatever experience or substance causes it. Empaths are often alcoholics, drug addicts, sex and love addicts, adrenaline junkies, overeaters, and gamblers. Some may have addictions that seem completely harmless on the surface, such as an obsession with crossword puzzles or addiction to buying new socks. It might sound silly, but even these "harmless" addictions can prove problematic for us, primarily because we use them as a way to shut out a part of ourselves when we ought to be learning to manage and embrace it.
- **We make friends fast maybe too fast** - This isn't usually a risky behavior when the bond is between two empathic types who are used to practicing reciprocity. But often, empaths who are

lonely or need to fill a void can form deep, intense bonds with new friends or lovers who lack similar empathetic capacity and these bonds seem to emerge virtually overnight. These relationships can become extremely intimate over a short period, perhaps because we as empaths are great at sensing or even anticipating the needs of others, and we can consistently provide precisely what the other person desires in a confidant, partner in crime, or source of entertainment. These relationships tend to burn bright but fizzle quickly, like fireworks, because they are mainly one-sided, with the empath doing the majority of the emotional labor. They also tend to involve poor or lopsided boundaries and other dynamics that are symptomatic of codependency.

- **We are not just tired; we are fatigued** - Many empaths suffer from conditions like lupus, chronic fatigue syndrome, or more commonly, anemia that persists in spite of an altered diet with high iron content. These conditions, coupled with our tendency to carry the emotional weight that shouldn't be ours to lug around, leaves many of us as exhausted after a dull day's work as someone who's just run a marathon. Sometimes, people misinterpret this fatigue and label us as lazy or unmotivated.
- **We have allergies** - Sensitive skin and delicate

stomachs are common for people like us. We often have to eat restricted diets and use organic, unscented toiletries. Some of us have to wear organic fabrics and hypoallergenic jewelry.

- **We don't always make good students or 9-to-5 employees** - Our emotional realities are still in flux, especially when we are in populated places like a school or office building. That means we can struggle with repetitive routines, strict rules, and controlling authorities that are all common in these environments. We feel trapped by these circumstances, frustrated by the impassivity of any institution that cannot bend the rules or alter schedules to accommodate the needs of the people within it. We usually thrive more in educational and career environments with a lot of freedom and frequent change, where emotional expression is highly valued, and timetables can be flexible.
- **We are not great with money** - There are two possible explanations for this reality. First, we can be erratic spenders who have trouble sticking to budgets; for an empath whose energy has been polluted by another person's trauma or despair, a bottle of wine or a banana split might feel like more than a mere craving. These sources of comfort seem like imperative purchases for us, as we fear that without them, we'd genuinely run the risk of spiraling out of control or exploding.

Secondly, we can be bad with money because the concept of capitalism is fundamentally at odds with our interior value system. Empaths feel guilty about accepting money from those whose needs they perceive to be greater or more important than their own (and sometimes, empaths perceive that group to consist of every single other person on the planet before themselves), and we are not comfortable with peacocking, tricks of salesmanship, or any form of dishonesty. Any empath who endeavors to start their own business would be wise to hire a financial consultant early in the process; otherwise, it may take them years to realize that they are mostly working for free.

- **We can be manipulated easily** - You'd think, with all the unspoken information we have access to, that empaths would be able to see through people with manipulative intentions. But alas, many of us are only attuned to emotion, so plans can be challenging to read, especially when strong feelings like excitement or fear overshadow them. Also, especially in youth, we want to see the best in people, and we might tie ourselves in knots so as not to acknowledge that someone is trying to use us.
- **When we care, we care too much** - Empaths tend to over promise ourselves; and then, since we are people pleasers and can't stand to let anyone

down, we over deliver in spades! This intensity of emotional generosity can sometimes put people off or scare them away, but we don't mean any harm by it.

- **But when we don't care, we couldn't care less** - Generally, empaths are not easily bored, as we have such a rich interior world to ponder at any given moment. But if we are given a job to complete that doesn't inspire passion in us, we will start to deflate like a balloon. We also have a very low tolerance for work that is morally compromising in any way, inefficient systems, and jobs that don't appear to have a reasonable, achievable end goal. In these situations, we usually disengage or slow down like a wind-up toy running out of batteries.

- **We know what's expected of us** - Even if the expectation isn't communicated, we have a talent for sensing when we're supposed to arrive early, right on time, or fashionably late. We can anticipate the way others will react to our behaviors and are used to quickly tailoring our presentations of self and expressions of opinion to manage potential consequences or reactions. This skill makes us excellent personal assistants, maids of honor or best men in wedding parties, musical accompanists to a main improvisational act, or event planners. It also

means we can appear quite paranoid and high-strung at times.
- **We have tender stomachs, and lower back pain** - Lower back problems and digestive disorders of all kinds are quite common amongst empaths. It may be because this is the location of the solar plexus chakra, Manipura, which is typically weak for us. (You'll find a more in-depth explanation of this, as well as the other chakras, later in the book.) Or, if you prefer an answer rooted in science rather than the metaphysical realm, this might be because humans tend to carry emotional tension in our back muscles, and manifest anxiety in our guts.
- **We carry extra weight in our stomachs** - This is a common trait of empaths, even those who exercise regularly and eat very healthily. It may be due, again, to our troubles with the 3rd chakra and inability to keep it balanced or unblocked. It also may be a result of the high levels of stress and anxiety we process, which can impact the body's ability to burn fat around the mid-section. We empaths also tend to hug or protect our abdomens while in the company of others, perhaps with a pillow or blanket or just thick, bulky clothing--particularly around people we do not trust.
- **We are water lovers** - Of course, loads of people love the ocean, and who doesn't enjoy a good

refreshing shower? For us, though, water is more than just a refresher or cleanser. This element has an immensely powerful influence over empaths; standing near the ocean, an empath might feel suddenly as respectful as a pilgrim reaching Mecca. Bathing is a transformative process for us; we often walk out of a shower feeling like an entirely new person. When we are dehydrated, our personalities change (and not for the better).

- **We are indecisive** - Generally speaking, we know what we like and dislike. But knowing what we want is an altogether different story. Empaths can agonize for hours over decisions that would only require a moment's consideration from the average person, like what shoes to wear or which brand of milk to buy. This is sometimes because our minds fixate more on the future than the present, and want to explore all the possible outcomes of any choice we make. We can also have episodes of paralyzing indecision when we are stuck in the mindset of seeking validation through the approval of others; in this state of mind especially, we can't distinguish between what we want, what others want for us, what others want from us, and what others want for themselves.
- **We are inquisitive** - Empaths are eager learners with an insatiable thirst for discovery and the pursuit of higher truths. Furthermore, when we are

charged with enough positive energy, we are excellent listeners and conversationalists--the type of people who would make great talk-show hosts. We ask nuanced questions because we are genuinely curious. We are often fascinated by that which seems mundane or uneventful to most people.

- **We are trusted** - For whatever reason, family, friends and strangers alike seem to want to confide in us. We hear a lot of sentences that begin with the words: "I've never told anybody about this before, but…" Generally, we are good at respecting privacy and keeping secrets, but it is odd that people can sense this without ever knowing about all the other secrets we've successfully kept to ourselves.
- **We have social lives like moon cycles** - An empath's social calendar is usually in a state of gradual flux--not quixotic or haphazard, but gently surging and receding like the phases of the moon. We tend to sway back and forth between wanting to be surrounded by other people's emotional energy, and needing total solitude, quiet and calm. It often takes us several days, or even a full week, to shift into a different phase.
- **We are easily distracted** - Left on their own in a controlled environment, empaths can stay focused on passion projects for long periods. But when an external stimulus is introduced, all bets are off. We

are not the best companions to take on a shopping trip if you have a limited amount of time, as we are likely to wander off when we catch sight of something shiny and get lost. Or worse, we'll get caught up in a deep discussion with an employee who's trying to sell us something we do not need. Please believe us when we tell you that we don't mean to be rude or throw your agenda off track. Sometimes, we really can't help it.

- **Yes, we hear, see, and smell everything** - Empaths are generally more sensitive than most, so odors, lights, colors, and sounds can sometimes seem harsh or abrasive to us, even when others hardly notice them. Some of us are extremely sensitive to touch, and even the sensation of wind against our skin is irritating. We can be great cooks because some of us can detect the specific herbs, spices, and flavor profiles used in anything we taste.
- **No, we can't just let it go** - Injustices don't just bother empaths--they shake us to our cores, whether the injustice is an insult to us personally or it has nothing to do with us at all. If something isn't done to remedy the inequity (whether that means the action isn't taken to right the wrong, or just that no remorse is expressed), the empath might feel that it is impossible to move on. In short, we recognize that sometimes, it is best to let go and cut our losses simply, but this theory is complicated for

us to put into practice. We can fall into spells of severe depression, obsessive-compulsive or manic episodes, especially if we convince ourselves that we can battle an injustice which, in reality, is far too high for us to face alone. We need close friends or lovers who can recognize these unhealthy thought patterns, exhibit patience, help us to see reason, and steer us back towards inner balance.

- **Our bodies are vessels** - And sometimes, we suspect them to be full of energy, emotion, and even personality traits that do not belong to us. During times of emotional stress or upheaval, an empath may feel an overwhelming sense of confusion about their behaviors. Looking in the mirror, an empath in distress might recoil, suddenly unable to recognize their reflection. We know firsthand how intense emotions can transform our physical bodies, and when we experience emotional contagion, it often shows in our facial features and posture, as well as through our habits. Emotions don't just affect us; they possess us like ghostly spirits.

- **We can read between the lines** - Empaths have a knack for picking up on the things people don't want to say out loud. We can tell when people are too bashful to flirt with each other. We can sense when a business is on the verge of collapsing. We can usually spot a scam from a mile away. And liars? They probably should steer clear of all empathic types. Nothing gets past us, and if people were not so emotional, we could be amazing detectives.

- **We feel genuine sympathy for the devil** - Empaths are often able to find both compassion and empathy for those people that society has mostly given up on or written off as beyond hope, such as violent criminals, child abusers, serial con artists, or pathological addicts. We don't necessarily believe their behaviors are excusable, but we can often see that they stem from a place of insecurity, fear, and deep emotional pain, rather than malice, and so our hearts go out to the victims buried deep inside of them. Meanwhile, non-empaths often see us as too forgiving, gullible, or idealistic to be rational. If the criminal justice system as a whole weren't such a volatile and inhospitable environment for our emotional energy fields, then we might make excellent public defense advocates. Empaths can recognize that some criminals may be guilty of perpetrating the crimes they are accused of, and still not be deserving of the standard punishment the system would choose for them. We are also hypersensitive to how the criminal justice system feeds into vicious cycles rather than interrupting them, frequently condemning people to lifelong careers of criminality rather than offering therapeutic pathways to change and positive growth.

- **We're at our best around children, animals, plants, and nature** - Children are more honest than adults. Dogs, cats, flowers, trees, and rocks never lie to us, either. Many empaths only feel at liberty to be fully themselves around these entities. Around other adults, we are always wearing some form of mask or shield to protect ourselves, and struggling to make sense of deception, cognitive dissonance, and unspoken tensions.
- **We are anachronisms** - Many empaths feel out of place in present-day society, and uncomfortable with the ubiquitous nature of modern technology. We are also often disconnected from our peers in our age group, preferring the company of those who are significantly older or younger than we are.
- **We follow the rules** - Especially in our younger years, empaths are goody-two-shoes types. We often behave as though we believe an authority figure is always watching us, even when we know we are alone. We are genuinely motivated by guilt and shame in childhood; as adults, we usually continue to make our decisions based on avoidance of punitive consequence, rather than on our true desires.
- **We are chameleons** - If we have the energy and desire to do so, we can fit in just about anywhere--

though it is exhausting. We'd make excellent spies, if only we weren't so sickened by violence and dishonesty.

- **We are walking contradictions** - Empaths embody dichotomies all the time. All at once, we might be happy and sad; calm, but livid with anger; idealistic, and yet profoundly cynical; childlike and naive, but with an old soul. It isn't always comfortable for us to carry such polarized emotions inside ourselves, but most of us are familiar with the feeling and find that though it can be painful, it helps to broaden our perspectives and enhances our empathic connection to other people.

4

Empath Types

By now, you may be feeling reasonably confident that you experience empathy to an atypical degree. But to hone and master your empathic skills, you'll need to determine what type of empath you are. Essentially, this is a question of what form of energetic vibration you pick up on the most easily.

The most common empath types are listed below. As you read, bear in mind that you might be a combination type-- perhaps you resonate with the experiences of both geomantic and animal empaths, or emotional and Claircognizant empaths. Maybe you are a combination of more than just two types. There are also some forms of empathy which are so rare as to be widely unrecognized, and these empath types often don't have official names.

While there are notable differences between them, all empath types are connected by a universal recognition of invisible forces and their effect on the physical world. As you enhance your sensitivity and strive towards spiritual expansion, you may discover new types of empathic connection within yourself. Stay open-minded.

Emotional Empaths

While the concept of empathy is difficult to measure, and it may be impossible to find accurate information on how many exist in our population today, it seems that emotional empaths are by far the most common type. It may be because of normal ranges of emotional empathy appearing present in most humans from birth. For most of us, the impulse to feel the emotions of others as deeply as our own weakens as we mature and develops a stronger sense of personal ego. Some of us, though, may hold onto these strong connections throughout our childhood, and then feel them even more powerfully as adults. Others may learn to bury their empathic feelings in adolescence, as peers put more and more pressure on them to toughen up and grow a thick skin, only to have their profoundly compassionate nature erupt with volcanic force at a later point in life. Many people discover their identities as emotional empaths through the breakdown of an emotionally unhealthy relationship.

Emotional empaths can feel the emotions of those who are

physically close to them. If they have friends, family, or lovers whom they come to know intimately, they can sometimes even sense their emotions across vast distances, through phone calls or emails. Some empaths may also be able to detect the feelings of the important people in their lives while they aren't in contact at all.

They are often keen at detecting energy shifts, even very minor ones. That is why emotional empaths can spot lies easily and are hard to keep secrets. They can usually feel unspoken group dynamics, or "vibes," and can sense the tension in other people's relationships, as well as sexual energy between others.

The emotional empath can often struggle to find a firm sense of self and maintain healthy boundaries in relationships. If you believe yourself to be a member of this group, you should take special care to avoid codependent behaviors with family members, lovers, and friends. Empaths may grow so accustomed to being full of the emotions of their loved ones, that they initially feel empty when left to their own devices. They also attract empathy-deficient types like flies to honey. Narcissists, in particular, can be very attractive to emotional empaths, who can benefit from the narcissist's nervous energy in two ways, at first; the empath can feel the same admiration for the narcissist that the narcissist thinks for themselves, and also feel emboldened by the narcissist's sense of confidence and lack of shame. This feeling of empowerment is intoxicating for the empath; it is usually fleeting, though, and often part of a cycle of abusive behavior that can have a truly corrosive effect on the empath's self-love and potential for future independence.

If you identify as an emotional empath, pay particular attention to any passages in the following chapters that mention boundaries and how to strengthen them. Emotions can shape our thoughts and our perceptions of life, so it is essential to take control of your emotional well-being. Learn how to recognize the relationships in your life that are emotionally unhealthy, how to minimize your exposure to emotional vampires, and how to deflect unnecessary negativity.

Physical Empaths

They are believed to be the second most common empathic type; physical empaths are also often referred to as medical empaths. While emotional empaths might share the psychological pain of those around them, the physical empath can share pains that stem from injury or illness. They may also share pleasant physical sensations that are experienced in the bodies of others, such as comfort, soothing massage, tickling, or sexual stimulation, but this seems to be less common than the detection of ailments and disease.

Some physical empaths might not feel the pain in another person's body; instead, they may merely see or sense the location of a disturbance or blockage in their energy field, stemming from an injury or illness that is invisible to the naked eye. This method is frequently used by empathic healers, practitioners of acupuncture, reiki, reflexology, and other non-western healing traditions.

For those who do share physical sensations, the impulse to work as a healer is something of a double-edged sword. Through exposure to so much discomfort, injury and sickness, the physical empath can take on enough symptoms to present as a patient with their chronic illness or autoimmune disease. They may find it frustrating or even fruitless to try and pursue a reliable diagnosis for the pains that plague them, as scans and tests will fail to detect any veritable causes.

Whether you wish to use your abilities to heal others, or merely want to navigate your way through life without aches and pains that aren't yours to bear, as a physical empath, you'll need to develop a strong energy shield. Learn to protect yourself before you attempt to cure other people. If you do become a healing practitioner of any sort, be sure to set aside plenty of alone time for yourself so that you can stay in touch with the feeling of your independent body, both in motion and at rest. Otherwise, you may run the risk of numbing yourself to your injuries or illnesses, unable to notice symptoms of your own before they grow deep roots and become difficult to treat.

Animal Empaths

Animal empaths appear to be reasonably rare. They are people who feel a stronger emotional or physical empathy towards animal species than they do with other humans.

Many animal empaths feel more comfortable in the company of any non-predatory animal species, and report that they can sense the needs and desires of animals. This ability often extends to multiple types of animals, but some empaths only have this strong connection with one group within the animal kingdom, with one specific species, or even with one individual animal. Some empaths seem to be able to locate or track animals in the wild more easily than most and are allowed to get closer to the native species than most humans would be. Very few empaths claim to have full telepathic connections with animals.

Most animals, especially those who live in packs, are natural empaths themselves. Without verbal communication, they have to be deeply sensitive to all the energetic dynamics around them for the sake of survival. Animals also lack awareness of many things that corrupt communication in human societies; they don't feel self-conscious about the size of their bank accounts or ashamed of their body shapes. The honesty of the animal ego coupled with their ability to love fully and unconditionally, makes time with animals refreshing and energizing for most empath types.

If you identify as an animal empath, it might be wise to

consider a vegan or vegetarian diet. If you must consume meat or animal products, aim to eat only those who are ethically sourced. This dietary change can have an enormous impact on your overall sense of well-being and inner balance. Some animal empaths report having such a strong connection to animal emotion as to be able to taste the fear of an animal slaughtered for meat. It is never a bad idea to try an elimination diet and get acquainted with the personalized needs of your digestive system; you may not even be aware of your food sensitivity until you try living a few weeks without meat or dairy, and realize you feel better than you ever have before.

If you don't already work with animals, you might want to spare a few hours on an upcoming weekend to visit or even volunteer at a local animal shelter. Use this time to check-in with yourself and evaluate whether or not this exposure to animal energy has a positive or negative effect on your emotional state. If so, it may be worth it to adopt a pet of your own or start volunteering regularly.

Plant Empaths

Plant empaths appear to be about as rare as animal empaths. They can sense the distinct needs of plants and trees; thus, they make excellent gardeners, farmers, and caretakers of nature reserves. The plant empath has a natural green thumb; they can coax seeds to thrive in environments where they usually might wither, and they can predict the fate of a crop earlier in its growth period than most almanacs could.

Even rarer still, some plant empaths have deep and powerful connections with ancient trees. They claim to receive messages and wisdom from them.

Plant empaths can become emotionally and physically uncomfortable when they are distanced from the natural world for long periods. If you identify as a plant empath, it's essential to fill your living space with live plants; think of caring for them as a part of your self-care routine, as they will generate a significant portion of the oxygen you breathe every day.

You may also want to make an effort to consume organic fruits, vegetables, and herbs--and very fresh ones, if possible. Sign up for a share of a local farm's crop yield, or patronize farmers markets whenever you can. Unlike animals, the primary purpose of all plants on this earth is to store and transform energy from the sun, so there is no need to feel any sense of guilt in consuming them if they are grown ethically. However, you might want to investigate the source of any product that is hard to find locally grown and organic; global consumer demand pushes some farmers to produce or distribute their crops in ways that negatively affect the surrounding environment. If you are particularly sensitive to plant energies, such a circumstance might present within you as an inability to digest the food in question, or a phantom sense of anxiety or depression after eating it.

The plant empath can often struggle to connect deeply with other humans. They might even resent humanity on a global level for the many forms of destruction we've levied against the natural world. As difficult as it might be, the plant empath should make an effort to reach beyond their comfort zone and foster connection with at least a handful of people, preferably some who share their deep concern for plant life. They might find it helpful to join an environmental organization to see such people while giving back to the natural world at the same time.

Geomantic Empaths

A geomantic empath has a genuinely phenomenal ability to pick up on the energetic vibrations of inanimate objects or inorganic materials. They are also sometimes referred to as environmental empaths.

Geomantic empaths generally fall into one of two categories. First, some are connected to individual objects, rooms or buildings, and can sense their histories. This type of geomantic empath will have extreme preferences for or aversion to previously owned clothing, household items, or cars, and can only live in buildings with happy emotional legacies.

The second type of geomantic empath maintains a connection to the earth itself, and all rocks and stones that were once a part of it, even the grains of sand on a beach or the microscopic minerals in salt or drinking water. These empaths can often detect impending natural disasters before any branch of science can predict them.

Both of these geomantic empath types tend to have heightened sensitivities to natural materials. Stone and rock, of course, but also wood (raw, petrified, or in any other state), hemp and linen, seashell and bone--these are all excellent materials to incorporate into your living space if you identify as a geomantic empath. You may also find that you reap even more significant benefits from crystal healing than most, so it's a great idea to fill your home with healing stones and lots of natural light. Grounding is also an excellent way for you to practice self-care, restore balance, and recharge, particularly near seashores, mountain ranges, or patches of earth that are undisturbed by modern architecture and technology.

History and art museums can be emotional rollercoasters for the geomantic empath, who feels deep connections to items and can be overwhelmed by the energetic charge of anything that's been on this planet for longer than the average human life-span.

Geomantic empaths are deeply connected to natural ecosystems, so they can find great joy through championing environmental causes. Join an organization that works to stop marine pollution or deforestation, or donate money to help sustain a nature reserve that is especially meaningful to you. You may also find you have a talent for designing homes or workspaces inspired by nature; you could easily thrive in the fields of green planning or organic design. Living in dense cities, or close to fault lines that cause frequent earthquakes and tremors, can ultimately have a destabilizing effect on you. They can disrupt your sense of inner balance.

Claircognizant Empaths

Also referred to as intuitive, claircognizant empaths can sense more about the people around them than their current emotional state or physical sensations. They pick up on energetic vibrations and frequencies, which sometimes allow them to receive specific messages about another person's past, future, or current circumstances beyond feelings. For instance, an emotional empath might meet someone new and sense only that the person is excited and happy, and the physical empath might share the feeling of butterflies in their stomach; the claircognizant empath, meanwhile, might be able to decipher that the cause of these sensations is a budding new romance. They can sometimes even pick up on more specific details, like the name or age of this person's new love.

Claircognizant empaths are quite rare, and those who do claim to possess this ability are, unfortunately, very often found to be frauds. If you are ever seeking assistance from a claircognizant empath, be very wary of those who appear to mass market their abilities, and especially those who adamantly pursue business from people in a state of grief or desperation.

If you identify as a claircognizant empath, be mindful of the fact that this rare gift comes with its fair share of risks and dangers. Reaching a state of emotional intimacy with others may prove to be a lifelong challenge for you, as you will struggle to recognize boundaries or to foster trust with others. If you choose to incorporate your empathic power into your career, be careful to maintain a balance between your work and your personal life, and don't allow your intuitive knowledge to lure you into a warped sense of confidence or invulnerability. No matter how strong your claircognizant power is, the world can always surprise you.

Medium Empaths

An empath may identify as a medium if they can sense or communicate with spirits who have passed away. They are also sometimes referred to as channels. Their powers most often work as a telephone wire, translating or transporting messages from a precisely defined source outside of the mortal or physical realm to interested parties here on earth. Occasionally, mediums can function as a surrogate body for a deceased entity, letting the spirit's voice, mannerisms, posture, and facial expressions flow throughout their bodies while the empath falls into a sort of black-out state.

No matter what form a medium receives messages in, their

gifts are extremely rare and often present very differently from one empath to the next. Some mediums can choose when and how they receive signals from the beyond, while others seem to receive messages at the whim of the spirits they commune with, whether their timing is convenient or not. Some mediums channel messages from the divine rather than from the deceased. The one definitive trait that all mediums share is the ability to source information from the immortal plane more easily than they can interpret messages from the living.

As with claircognizant empathy, there are unfortunately many con artists and frauds who falsely claim to possess this type of power and use these feigned abilities for the sake of personal financial gain, at the expense of believers and right mediums in turn. If you genuinely can sense energy or messages from the deceased, there is nothing wrong with offering assistance to those grieving the loss of a loved one; furthermore, there is nothing wrong with asking for adequate payment, since channeling this energy can be quite physically and emotionally taxing for the empath. However, everyone should be wary of mediums who pursue clients, knowing they are in grief or otherwise emotionally vulnerable.

Many mediums find the experience of channeling all-encompassing and immensely exhausting. If you identify as a medium empath, you have likely already learned to be careful about which spirits you allow to use your body and mind as a channel. Corruption or possession by malicious spirits is a severe risk, and since there are so few empaths and healers in the world who are equipped to eradicate such afflictions, you are better off avoiding the possibility entirely. Stick with spirits that you feel comfortable with, and trust in your gut instincts. Be ready to disconnect any channel the instant you sense the threat of danger.

Precognitive Empaths

A precognitive empath is attuned to the energetic vibrations of the future. Most, however, do not claim to have any clear or precise predictions of days to come, and they often have very little control over how and when they receive information. A large number of precognitive empaths receive their empathic knowledge through dreams or visions, and the information they see is usually abstract or symbolic. Some precognitive empaths receive information while awake, but again, they are often the only privy to a general sense of foreboding or dread before a catastrophe, rather than being granted the precise information needed to prevent the disaster or adequately warn others — some sense future happenings primarily through strong repetitive feelings of deja vu or phantom anxieties.

Precognitive empaths may find that the ancient myth of Cassandra resonates deeply with their experience, eloquently illustrating how their empathic gift can be as much of a curse as it is a blessing. In this myth, Cassandra was at first a mortal princess; the god Apollo fell in love with her from afar, and approached her, hoping to win her affections by offering her the godly power of prophetic foresight. Cassandra accepted the gift at first and agreed to be his paramour, but then changed her mind. Furious, Apollo layered a curse atop her supernatural gift; henceforth, Cassandra would see the future, but no matter how she tried to warn others of what was coming, no one would ever believe her. Eventually, people came to think of her as insane.

Similarly, precognitive empaths are likely accustomed to having their claims dismissed or disbelieved. Many even grow deeply discouraged by the opinions of non-believers, and give up on their gifts, distancing themselves from their prophetic knowledge on purpose. Like any form of empathy, precognitive ability it not fixed; it can be nourished and strengthened or starved and weakened. If you identify as a precognitive empath and wish to enhance your skills, an excellent place to start is with regular dream journaling. The more frequently and diligently you record the abstract symbols and messages you come across in your dreams, the more likely you are to notice patterns or important details that stand out.

For the sake of your peace of mind, you may want to take proactive steps to combat or prevent symptoms of anxiety. Figure out what forms of meditation, aromatherapy, or sonic healing work best to keep you calm and level-headed.

You may also be more likely than most to carry your concerns about the future in your stomach and upper digestive tract, suffering from conditions such as acid reflux or stomach ulcers. An elimination diet can be helpful, and you may find relief through cutting out coffee, cigarettes and soft drinks. You can also channel focused, positive energy to your 5th chakra, vishuddha, at the base of your throat, allowing you to communicate your precognitive wisdom to others better. Your third eye chakra is likely to be hyperactive already, so favor practices that balance this chakra over those that seek to open it further.

5

Benefits, drawbacks, and dangers of empathic power

It should be clear by now that heightened empathy can be both a positive and negative trait. Here, we'll first explore the reasons why you might be grateful for and excited by your empathic ability. Then, we'll outline some of the frustrations empaths commonly share; and lastly, we'll describe some of the risks that empaths should be very careful to avoid.

First, the good

There are many benefits to be found in empathic power of any type or level of strength.

Empaths feel emotional responses to intense degrees, so when they are happy, they are over the moon. When they feel loved and supported, they are downright giddy. When they get excited about a new idea, they become determined and powerful enough to move mountains.

They are easily moved and may derive more sheer pleasure from entertainment and artistic media than most people.

Empaths are also great soothsayers, which can make them very useful therapists, salespeople, emergency responders, or administrators in emotionally turbulent fields--working in the neonatal wing of a hospital. For instance, an empath might be especially adept at helping patients to feel calm and understand what's happening with their infants. This talent does not come without a price, however--empaths can be great at promoting relaxation in other people, but this practice is often emotionally and physically taxing.

They can sense danger and volatile energy, so empaths have an easier time than most in escaping risky situations before things get out of hand.

Empathy, in general, motivates altruistic behavior, so empaths are often driven to help others in a truly selfless way. Whereas many people make charitable donations or volunteer for self-serving reasons, either hoping to be seen as virtuous or to restore personal faith in their proper nature after a moral failing, empaths are driven by the earnest belief that they help themselves whenever they help others, or furthermore, that they help everyone when they help anyone. Empaths make incorruptible leaders, as they can remove the influence of their ego from the equation and focus all of their energy on the greater good.

Empaths are great problem solvers because they can examine conflicts from multiple perspectives, explore the nuance, and suggest resolutions that involve mutual compromise. They can help steer adversaries away from the blame game, usually acknowledging that there are faults on both sides of any argument, and keeping them focused instead on progress and forward momentum.

Finally, empaths don't need much in the way of stimulation to feel contented or well-entertained. They are often able to make the most of situations that others might find torturously dull. They can also thrive within minimalist environments, and sustain healthy long-distance relationships with minimal opportunity for contact, and can easily access feelings of excitement without the stimulus of novelty or pandemonium.

Then, the bad

Empaths can be indecisive to the point of absurdity. They often struggle to make major or minor decisions because they can see or feel an overwhelming number of possible outcomes to whatever choice they make.

Time management can be a serious struggle for empaths.

Empaths may find it nearly impossible to stick to any form of rigid schedule or meet strict deadlines.

Loud noises, big crowds, unpleasant odors, and bright lights--these are all certain aspects of modern life, especially if you live in a major city. But empaths can have a very low tolerance for these things, meaning the outside world can sometimes seem like one enormous synesthetic minefield to them. Depending on their energy reserves and self-care routines, the empath may sometimes feel too anxious or frightened to leave the security and predictability of their own home for days, even if this self-imposed imprisonment works to their ultimate detriment.

Empaths can be extraordinarily self-conscious or even paranoid at times. They might pick up on "bad vibes" from a friend or colleague, and then twist themselves in knots trying to understand why this person won't confront or acknowledge the discord between them. They note subtle displays of passive aggression and wish that they could respond with a direct invitation to hash things out, though most have learned that a gesture like this rarely fosters a positive resolution.

It can be challenging for the empath to come to terms with the fact that their sensitivities are uncommon, and that therefore, it may not be possible to share the depth of their own experience with most others. Many grow up believing that all people see, hear, and feel the world in the same way that they do, especially if others do not validate their sensitivities during childhood. They may suffer from the belief that others carry just as heavy an emotional or energetic load as them, and other people are naturally better at managing it gracefully. It can be jarring to realize later in development that some are truly blind, deaf, or numb to the sensations the empath finds impossible to ignore, and furthermore, to discover just how many adults purposefully distance themselves from their emotions like a permanent coping strategy. Empaths often struggle with emotional intimacy, as there is a very narrow section of the population that is well-suited to the depth of emotional connection that comes naturally to highly sensitive people.

Boundaries can be difficult for empaths to manage. They often struggle to establish and maintain their own, as well as to recognize and respect the boundaries of people they love. For instance, an empath may sense that a friend is sad, but if this emotion hasn't been verbally conveyed, their offer to help may come across as pushy or invasive. It can make emotional intimacy challenging. Empaths may identify with the story of Goldilocks in close relationships; they are always either too open and available, or also closed off and distant, but they rarely feel like they are getting it just right.

Empaths also tend to be engulfed in intimate relationships, and can quickly start to lose their sense of self as it is overshadowed by or entangled with the identity of their companion. That means break-ups can be excruciating, as the empath feels that they are losing a part of themselves along with their departing lover.

And now, the ugly

People with typical ranges of empathy have sensitivities that don't require much maintenance. But those with true empathic powers must take ownership of their abilities, educate and train themselves to manage their empathy. If you identify as an empath, embrace the fact that you are on a lifelong journey with slight upward incline and no apex in sight. No matter how enlightened you become, your sensitivity will never be able to self-regulate or self-sustain without your attentive guidance. Without this vigilant attitude, empathic power can become a destructive force. The empath should never lose sight of this fact, lest their powers grow vulnerable to corruption.

Empaths and narcissists seem complicated, maybe even cosmically, linked. Some might like to believe that narcissists are to blame, preying on vulnerable empaths--but the truth is, both parties bear responsibility for this abusive dynamic. Empaths often blind themselves to the negative aspects of a narcissist's personality and support the belief that the narcissist's thoughts and feelings are more important than the empath's, or anyone else's, for that matter. Without purposeful training of their empathic abilities, they are likely to become codependent in these relationships, feeding into the cycle of emotional abuse rather than working towards healing.

An empath who has not yet been awakened or enlightened to their gift can grow to become a tragic figure. Without awareness of the fact that empaths are beacons for empathy deficient personalities and broken, wounded souls, they may spend their entire lives surrounded by people who only take from their energy reserves, and never give back a drop. That can leave the empath feeling embittered and resentful of their loved ones, or of humanity at large, when they begin to notice that their personal needs are being ignored while others are taken care. There are some who believe this is the root of narcissism--a failed or reformed empath may reach a breaking point and decide that the only way to have their needs met is to mimic the behaviors of those who have used the empath as a healer and then promptly tossed them aside.

Finally, for those with extremely advanced empathic sensitivity, the mind can become hyperactive and draw energy from the body, or vice versa. A physical empath with deep sensitivity might eventually become so rooted in their pains and physical sensations as to lose their mental capacities. Conversely, a precognitive empath might become consumed by their preoccupation with the future, and eventually forget to take care of their physical body, starving it, ignoring to sleep or exercise, or in very extreme cases, even falling into a coma.

These points are not outlined to motivate you through fear, but rather to remind you that empathy is fluid energy. It is neither inherently good nor bad. Your experience will depend entirely on how well you manage your energy flow. In the next few chapters, you'll find plenty of outlined strategies to help you enhance the beneficial aspects of your power, minimize the challenges, and avoid significant risks.

6

Making the Most of it

In this chapter, you'll be guided through your first few steps of a spiritual journey that will help you to thrive with your empathic abilities. No matter what type of empath you are, some basic practices can always serve to restore your dynamic balance and strengthen your sense of self. Pick and choose the methods that work best for you, or incorporate all of them into your routine if possible.

Purposeful Isolation

Sadly, a large number of empaths only come to discover their sensitivities when they are abandoned by the empathy-deficient people in their lives, usually in early adulthood. Some describe this experience as a reckoning or rite of passage for empaths; others might describe it as hitting rock bottom before ascending towards enlightenment. Once left on their own, they finally begin to understand the depths of their unmet emotional needs, feeling lonely, unspeakably depleted or used, misunderstood and undervalued. It is a painful way to come to such a revelation, so if you suspect you are an empath yourself, it may be wise to take a proactive approach, seeking out loneliness on your terms before it finds you unwilling and unprepared.

Empaths tend to put everyone else's needs before their own, and often develop hectic, busy lifestyles in adolescence to justify their volatile mood swings and unexplained anxieties. If this is true for you, then scheduling a significant stretch of solo time for yourself might feel awkward, undeserved, or even a bit frightening. Try to push through your apprehensions and plan a self-care retreat. Aim to schedule an extended period--ideally a full day or longer--to clear your energetic field of all pollution from other people, and get back in touch with yourself.

If money and time are no object, then a great way to do this is to plan a solo vacation. Bodies of water, especially the ocean, can give empaths a tremendous amount of therapeutic energy, so beaches and lakeshores make fantastic travel destinations. Be wary of major tourist spots, though, and remember that many people travel to escape their troubles, carrying suffering and negative energies with them. They may be able to drown out their own painful emotions with alcohol, adrenaline rushes, and other indulgences, but that won't stop you from picking up on their inner turmoil. For this retreat, you'd be wise to avoid tourist spots and peak hours.

Camping is another great way to connect with nature as you restore your inner balance. If safety is a concern for you, you might instead plan a couple of day hikes and spend the nights secure in a motel or travel vehicle, behind locked doors. Yoga, meditation, and spa retreats also make fantastic destinations, if you prefer more structure in your vacation plans.

Of course, the cost of traveling and demands of our careers prevent most of us from planning vacations at the drop of a hat, but there's still plenty that you can do to reconnect with your root energy and find balance with two days alone, in your home and neighborhood. The point of this exercise is to break your routine and distance yourself from the energy fields that frequently bleed into your own. You don't necessarily need to spend a lot of money to do this.

To get the most out of this practice, you'll want to minimize screen time, contact with friends, co-workers and loved ones, and intoxication through alcohol or illegal drugs. If you are accustomed to a busy lifestyle, you may want to schedule an itinerary for yourself as a strategy to prevent anxiety. Or, if you are feeling ready for an intense reckoning, leave the time open, start with quiet, reflective meditation, and allow your thoughts to cascade without limit. It might be an intensely emotional experience, so there's no shame in feeling overwhelmed, needing to cut the retreat short, or reaching out to a loved one for support. Still, try to remember that pain is a part of growth here. You can delay the experience or soften the blow, but you cannot outrun it or avoid it forever. Through isolation, you are finding your true self. Take it from an empath who has lived through such a reckoning; your evolution is worth the temporary discomfort.

Meditation

Meditation is a natural and logical next step for an empath. It can be very uncomfortable, at first, to sit quietly, all alone with your thoughts. Try to remember that the purpose of meditation is to let those thoughts and emotions come, and then release them. Allow them to wash over you the way waves move over your feet when you walk along the seashore, crashing up and then quickly, gently, fading away.

You can also meditate on specific subjects or questions that you struggle to comprehend. The purpose of meditation is not to stir anxiety, though, so if you note repetitive, obsessive, or negative thought patterns, you may want to change your approach before your next session.

If you are already well-practiced in meditation, you might want to challenge yourself further and awaken your third eye chakra by challenging your thought patterns. Some spiritual guides suggest using inquisition to aid this process, continually answering each of your thoughts with the question: "Is that true?" If that method feels combative or sparks feelings of internal conflict, you can instead practice disbelieving your thoughts, entertaining the possibility that the truth is the opposite of what you perceive it to be.

Create a Safe Haven

To ensure that self-care becomes a regular part of your new routine, you'll want to make space for it in your life--literally. Even if it has to be inside a closet, make sure you find some space to create a haven for yourself. You could also think of it as a peace bubble, meditation space, or a holy altar. The idea is to create an ideal space in which to center yourself whenever life outside this haven starts to feel overwhelming. You may want to fill it with candles and crystals, smudge sticks, plants, cozy pillows, and blankets. If you relish the endless potential of a blank slate, your haven might be completely bare, dark and quiet. There is no right or wrong way, only the way that feels right for you.

De-clutter and Organize your Living Space

Now that you've created a haven, your next goal should be to arrange the rest of your living space in a way that helps you to feel balanced, organized, efficient, and at peace. Even if you don't consider yourself a visual or materially-oriented person, the way your home looks matters; it is the first thing your eyes see every morning when you wake up, and the last thing you see before you fall asleep at night. Its appearance makes a mark on your dreams and the subconscious world, as well as on your conscious thought processes. Furthermore, the way it smells, sounds, and feels is meaningful, too.

If you find the theories of feng shui resonate with you, then go ahead and evaluate the layout of your home and furniture, and rearrange whatever you have to respect its principles. This is especially recommended for geomantic empaths--feng shui is also sometimes called "geomancy," and it addresses the same energetic frequencies that geomantic empaths are attuned.

If there's no time for a full interior redecoration effort, then instead, you may want to focus on clearing unwanted energy from your living space. Take a mental inventory of the items on display in your home. How many of them were items you chose based on desire? How many did you want based on necessity? Be on the lookout for gifts you've received, and remind yourself that you are alone and no one is judging you before you ask yourself: how do I feel about these items that were given to me? Do they have sentimental value and represent a feeling of love and affection for me? Or, were some of them provided by people who were trying to manipulate or influence my behaviors? Do some of them remind me that people in my life don't get me or understand who I am?

If so, don't feel ashamed for acknowledging it. Sometimes, gifts are not given from a place of generosity, but in an attempt to exert willpower. Recognize these items in your home as centers of negative or stagnant energy, and give yourself permission to dispose of them, give them away, or send them to remote storage.

Yoga, Tai Chi, and Physical Mindfulness Practice

Exercise is undoubtedly good for the body and soul, but it can be even more effective when combined with mindfulness. Mindfulness is the concept of heightening our awareness of things we usually take for granted or have learned to ignore, like our breathing or thought patterns. Yoga is especially popular, as it addresses the need for physical alignment and mindfulness, promoting focus, relaxation, acceptance, and self-love. It can also be tailored easily to suit many different needs, sometimes fully embracing its spiritual element, or at other times being exclusively concerned with the physical body. You can easily find a yoga class to attend, and there are many schools of yoga to choose from, depending on your desire to enhance strength, find balance, repair injury, or find more profound relaxation. You can also practice alone in your home, our outdoors in nature.

Tai chi also stimulates mindfulness through a series of slow, controlled physical movements. Generally, yoga can pose more of a physical challenge, whereas Tai chi requires a great deal of patience and focus, so it challenges the mind. It also looks more like a dance form, so those who feel freed by creative expression may prefer tai chi to other similar practices.

Grounding

Grounding is theoretically secure, but will only be as effective as the amount of energy you channel into the practice. All you need to do is remove your shoes and socks, plant your feet on the ground (ideally in a place where you feel a strong connection to nature) and imagine you are growing roots like a tree. Many empaths will close their eyes, breathe deeply, and utilize some form of meditation or affirmation during their grounding practice.

One mantra that you might find useful is the alternating repetition of two phases: first, "I am one with the universe," where you may substitute the word "universe" with "all things" or the name of a higher power in your faith; and secondly, "I am distinct, unique, powerful and purposeful." These two phrases articulate polarized sentiments that many empaths mentally seesaw back and forth between; the goal here is to honor both ideas as part of the same universal truth.

Some empaths find this practice especially powerful near oceans, historical landmarks, or sites of natural phenomena, like volcanoes or earthquakes. Grounding is highly recommended for geomantic and precognitive empaths.

Dietary Changes

Every living being, whether plant, animal or human, is made of energy. So if you are consistently consuming foods that carry forms of negative energy, it can manifest in your body as chronic pain, illness, malnourishment, or even as an emotional symptom, like depression.

An elimination diet is a simple way to effect significant change in your energy field, and it usually provokes rapid change. You may be shocked to find aches or points of tension are suddenly released, even though you never also noticed them before they were flushed away.

Intermittent fasting can also be a useful tool to enhance mental clarity, though it should be done with caution. Those who lead highly active lifestyles or suffer from nutritional imbalances may find this practice dangerous.

Affirmations and Manifestation Exercises

Have you ever had the experience of feeling overwhelmed by a mental to-do list, only to write it out on paper or tell someone else about it, and suddenly realize that it's easily doable, and not worth stressing?

Or, have you ever felt that a dream or wish was too far out of reach to entertain--but then, by declaring it aloud, you suddenly felt it drawn closer to you, entirely within reach?

This is a manifestation in action. Whether you intend to address it or not, the universe is listening to you, so proclaiming your desires and self-esteem clearly can have a fantastic ripple effect on your life. It can amplify your confidence, strengthen your resolve, encourage feelings of gratitude, and help you to maintain positive energy. Just be sure to project your truth without distortion, and be careful not to ask the universe for anything you aren't prepared to receive.

Use verbal or written affirmations during any self-love practice (yoga, meditation, bathing, or even while getting dressed in the morning, if you are pressed for time) to drive motivation, encourage self-love, and stay focused on your personal goals and values. Manifestation will be more focused on the future, whereas affirmations influence your current perceptions of reality. Remember that our thoughts shape our realities, so the simple act of reframing negative thoughts through the language of gratitude can change your entire outlook on life.

Journaling

There is no right or wrong way to use this practice. Regular free-writing is a fantastic way to find greater clarity of thought, as well as to self-soothe unexpressed frustrations or concerns. It may also be helpful to read over past entries from time to time, like a detective, whenever you suspect interference from a phantom source of negativity in your energy field. Journaling will help you to note healthy and risky patterns in your behavior, as well as within the framework of your interpersonal relationships. It will also be cathartic, helping you to let go of negative feelings and leave them sealed in the past.

7

Protecting the Empathic Self through
ENERGY HEALING

If you have subjected yourself to guided meditations or yoga practices or worked with any metaphysical healer, it's highly likely that you're already familiar with chakras. Unfortunately, many of us hear about chakras in passing without ever being educated on their basic definitions, let alone learning how to keep them open, balanced, and healthily functioning. Here, we'll outline the basics of chakra cleansing for all people, with a particular focus on the chakras that tend to need the most attention and care in empathic individuals.

Basics of energy healing

The word "chakra" comes from the Sanskrit word for

"wheel." Chakras are centers of energy within the body; working in synchronized concert, each is an energetic spinning vortex (hence the terminology) that governs the function of everything inside us, from our organs and immune systems to our interior emotional landscapes. There are seven chakras commonly recognized in the human body, each falling along the line that runs from the crown of the head, straight down to the root chakra at the base of the spine. Each one has its energetic frequency, its resonating color, and its form of energetic vibration. Some imagine them as whirlpools of energy that serve as portals to higher realms.

In any discussion about chakras, you are also likely to hear the words "kundalini" and "reiki" thrown around a great deal. Kundalini is a Hindu term for the spiritual energy or vital life force that each of us carries within. It is also sometimes called "the sleeping goddess" inside who must be awakened, or it may be referred to as "serpent power" because it is frequently illustrated as a resting snake, tightly coiled around the root chakra, at the base of the spine. Kundalini is also often imagined as a physical manifestation of energetic vibration. Many people envision it as a viscous, liquid light that can rise from the first chakra and illuminate the other six energy centers in the body as it passes them by.

Kundalini awakening is a challenging process. Those who are not adequately prepared for this spiritual journey may find themselves overwhelmed, deeply confused, or disoriented, needing to take a few steps back to the basics with increased discipline before attempting to raise their kundalini again. You may benefit from kundalini yoga, which is specially designed to awaken and enhance this raw form of energy. You must also remember to stay humble and open to learning from those who have walked this path before you, seeking wisdom from experienced healers. Since energetic vibrations vary so widely from one person to the next, there are no one-size-fits-all written guides to raising kundalini; therefore, meeting a teacher or guide in person is the best way to advance this spiritual practice.

Reiki is a Japanese tradition of energy healing. It can be used to address sources of physical discomfort, emotional turmoil, or both at the same time. Though the concepts of chakra work and reiki originated in different parts of the world during different historical periods, they have a great deal in common and are often both embraced by metaphysical healers, sometimes used in combination with one another to channel even more powerful healing energies.

In Reiki tradition, vital life force is referred to as "ki," and centers of this energy within the body are called "tandens" rather than "chakras." Reiki recognizes only three tandens in the human body--one in the center of the forehead, one in the middle chest above the rib cage, and finally, one in the lower abdomen beneath the navel, with the last tanden being considered the most important of the three. Reiki also works towards a form of spiritual awakening, though it is perhaps more accessible than kundalini; anyone who wishes to become awakened to Reiki energy needs only to seek out a master for a Reiki initiation, after which point they will be able to use Reiki for their own healing needs.

Many healers view chakra work and reiki work as two interpretations of the same idea, recognizing both kundalini and ki as the same spiritual energy force, just called by different names. The tandens and chakras all fall within the same physiological line, and when negative energy blocks or distorts the function of any organ or muscle in this area, vigorous metaphysical healing efforts will need to be applied; otherwise, illness, discomfort, and negative emotions will be able to thrive and fester inside, preventing your unique personal energy from flowing freely.

If you are someone who doesn't believe in spiritual healing arts, you may be ready to skip past this chapter--but I hope you'll read on, even if you typically only respect western medicine's take on the human body. It might interest you to know that the seven chakras closely mirror our endocrine systems, which are comprised of the glands that determine hormone release into our bloodstreams and govern every aspect of our growth and behavior, from emotion to metabolism and energy levels. Whether you incorporate crystals, smudging sticks, and shamanic guides in your healing practice, or opt to work with just your body and a yoga mat, it is always a good idea for empaths to get in touch with their chakras and reflect on how each is genuinely feeling. In our progress oriented society, everyone feels pressure to display constant forward momentum and charge ahead at a mile a minute. Stop, take a deep breath, and break the routine; set aside some time to listen to your body.

The seven major chakras

There are also minor chakras, but the seven major chakras are most commonly referenced in metaphysical healing. However, if you are a geomantic empath, you may want to explore the twelve chakra system, as the minor chakras focus more on our connection to the earth.

It's important to keep in mind that each of the seven (or twelve) is meant to function as a part of the whole system. Injury or imbalance to one chakra should never be ignored, as, over time, it will inevitably impact the healthy function of the others. Likewise, repairing the root chakra can have a positive domino effect on all your other chakras in turn, restoring overall balance from the bottom up; the same can be said of the crown chakra, dispersing divine energy to all the chakras beneath it.

First Chakra

The first, which we've already mentioned above, is the root chakra, or Muladhara, located at the base of the spine. Its resonant color is bright, vibrant red, and a lotus flower symbolizes it with four petals. Its element is earth. The root chakra is connected to blood circulation, the function of the feet and legs, spinal column, teeth, and the skeleton as a whole. This is where we house our feelings about our families and tribal affiliations (which, in modern day terms, may translate to political allegiances, social circles, ethnic or cultural backgrounds, etcetera.), as well as our emotions about finance. It is heavily tied to feelings of safety, security, and stability. This is where the fight or flight instinct stems from.

The root chakra may be firmly rooted and balanced within a person who does not need to worry about their basic needs (food, water, shelter, love) being met consistently. Conversely, a person who was raised in an environment where these securities were not always accessible may suffer from a chronic imbalance of the root chakra, even long after they have found stability by changing their life circumstances.

When an individual has an imbalanced or blocked root chakra, this can present through psychological symptoms like anxiety disorders, irrational fears, and repeated night terrors; it can also show through physical discomfort or malfunction in the bladder, lower digestive tract, legs and feet. Emotionally, this person may feel stuck in a rut, depressed, incapable of reaching their goals, or full of unexplained fear. The root chakra is the foundation of all other energy centers in the body, so with it weakened or imbalanced, it makes sense for a person to feel afraid or unmotivated. Working to restore kundalini in this area is always a great first step in metaphysical healing.

Second Chakra

Next is the sacral chakra, Svadhishthana, which is found below the navel. Its resonant color is orange, and its symbol is a lotus with six petals and three divine circles inside, layered to represent the phases of the moon. Its element is water. This chakra is where we source our emotional, creative, and sensual energies. It governs the function of our reproductive organs, as well as kidney function. The sacral chakra is where we hold feelings of desire; it can become imbalanced or blocked by a stifling of sexual energy, but also by an overabundance of it.

Your sacral chakra may be blocked if you're feeling pessimistic, creatively stuck, or if you seem to be encountering the same problems in relationships over and over again. You may feel lazy and unmotivated, underappreciated or unwanted, and your libido may be unusually low. Conversely, a person with an overactive sacral chakra may present as anxious, aggressive, full of themselves, and emotionally needy. Either form of imbalanced energy needs to be centered on improving your relationships and reconnecting with your sensory desires.

Third Chakra

The solar plexus chakra, Manipura, resides in the center of the stomach. Its resonant color is sunshine yellow, and its symbol is a ten-petaled lotus. Its element is fire. This chakra controls many major organs, including the liver, pancreas, all digestive organs, lungs, and adrenal glands. It is where we house personal ego, willpower, self-esteem, and confidence in our abilities. It is also where we store and process our emotions.

Many empaths struggle to keep their solar plexus balanced, open, and properly energized. This chakra often becomes impaired in victims of emotional or physical abuse. When the solar plexus chakra is malfunctioning, emotional turmoil rules the entire body. If you have a blockage or imbalance here, it can present as constant self-doubt or confusion, feelings of powerlessness or incompetence, and chronic frustration. Unfortunately, it can be hard to identify this blockage through symptoms alone, since they sometimes present as opposites; you might exhibit extremely low self-esteem, or an inflated ego, depending on which way this imbalance is skewed. Your skin might feel very hot to the touch, or very cold. Both are symptoms of the same problem, two sides of the same coin.

It can be very uncomfortable to house a malfunctioning solar plexus chakra, as it is linked to so many major interconnected organs. That being the case, a person with an impaired third chakra is likely to seek comfort in indulgence and vice and may suffer from substance addiction, hoping to numb themselves to their inner pain.

Fourth Chakra

The heart chakra, Anahata, sits in the center of the chest. Its resonant color is bright green, and its symbol is a lotus with twelve petals. Its element is air. This chakra is responsible for your heartbeat, blood circulation, and air flow to the lungs. It serves to connect the upper and lower chakras, and when it is healthy, it helps to provide a sense of serenity and balance. A person with an open heart chakra can trust, and can both give and receive unconditional love.

In Sanskrit, the word "Anahata" translates as: "unhurt, unstruck, unbeaten." Its energy relates to love and interpersonal connection on an emotional rather than sensual level. When this chakra is blocked, bitterness, resentment, and loneliness reign. This blockage may also present as chronic social anxiety. This chakra can be thrown off balance by heartbreak, rejection, or abusive relationship dynamics.

Fifth Chakra

The throat chakra, Vishudda, rests at the base of the throat. Its resonant color is aquamarine, or light blue, and its element is akasha (which translates as space, aether, or sky--a cosmic portion). Its symbol is a lotus flower with sixteen petals; each petal represents one of the sixteen vowel sounds in the Sanskrit language. This chakra is our center of communication and expression, and it regulates the function of the thyroid, esophagus, and vocal cords.

An individual with a poorly functioning throat chakra will have problems with speech. They might lie or omit truths; they might speak too quietly, or become aggressively talkative, dominating conversations. They might develop a stutter or other speech impediment; alternatively, they might present this blockage through an inability to listen attentively. The throat chakra also governs non-verbal expression, so an imbalance could prompt body language or artistic expression that seems to contradict the words or intentions they are paired with.

Like the solar plexus, the throat chakra is commonly blocked or impaired in empaths. This may be because society teaches empaths to swallow so many of their emotional experiences and become comfortable holding unspoken truths inside for years.

Sixth Chakra

The third eye chakra, Ajna, can be found at the center of the forehead, just above the eyes. Its element is light, and its resonant color is indigo. The symbol for this chakra is a lotus with only two petals and an inverted triangle within a perfect circle, mimicking the shape of a human eye. It is where the energies of intuition, wisdom, and spiritual enlightenment are sourced within the body. This chakra is connected to the eye, ear, brain, pituitary and pineal glands.

Whereas most will describe other chakras as blocked or functioning, balanced or imbalanced, the third eye is typically considered closed (though still energetically active) from birth until an individual reaches a point of spiritual awakening, at which point the third eye begins to open. When this chakra is awakened and in good health, the feminine and masculine energies within an individual become balanced, and they often find it easier to detach from material concerns.

Whether closed or open, this chakra can still function, or fall into imbalance. The third eye with insufficient energy flow might leave you confused, forgetful, unfocused, and afraid of anything you do not fully understand. On the other hand, too much energy flowing to this chakra can overstimulate spiritual power, causing mania and even hallucinations. Physical symptoms of an imbalanced third eye might include insomnia, high blood pressure, and migraines.

Seventh Chakra

The crown chakra, Sahasrara, rests at the uppermost point of the head, atop the skull. Its resonant color is violet purple, or sometimes white with a hint of lavender, and its element is consciousness or spirit. While the root chakra connects us to the earth, the crown chakra keeps us connected to the energy of the cosmos. This chakra shares dominion over the pituitary and pineal glands with the third eye chakra. It also governs the nervous system.

This chakra has a great deal in common with its neighbor, the third eye, but the crown is further removed from personal ego, focused on higher consciousness, universal truths, and connection to the limitless divine.

The most common symptoms of crown imbalance are cynicism and self-righteous, closed-minded belief. It might be triggered by an episode of spiritual disillusionment or general lack of exposure to spiritualism. Too little energy in this area can cause depression, pessimism, feelings of insignificance or belief that humanity is somehow doomed. Too much power, on the other hand, can lead a person's kundalini to reside only in mind, leaving the body behind to wither.

Chakra healing

Root Healing

Imbalance in the root chakra reflects a reluctance to trust in the universe, or any other higher power, to take care of your individual needs. Working to open, unblock, or balance this chakra means seeking to embody the same state of mind that animals occupy each day, never knowing where they'll find their next meal or which corners danger lurks behind, but still always moving forward, living in the present rather than fearing the unknown future or trying to control it.

Meditation is the simplest way to restore healthy energy in this area because of it both grounds you and connects you spiritually to a higher plane, at the same time. The root chakra is also linked to your sense of smell, so focusing energy at the tip of your nose during meditation can help to foster correct alignment in this part of the body. Since the color red is strongly correlated to the root chakra, crystals like garnet, red jasper, or bloodstone can be placed over the tailbone during yoga or other healing practices to help open and cleanse the area.

You can also employ the root chakra's corresponding mantra sound, lam, in combination with some yoga poses that are well-suited to root grounding work, such as mountain pose (tadasana) or garland pose (malasana).

Sacral Healing

You'll note that meditation and yoga are recommended for healing any of the seven chakras. For the sacral chakra, in particular, you may want to meditate on the nature of sensual pleasure, using yellow crystals like citrine in your practice. Moonstone will also resonate with this chakra's energy, due to its close relation to both the moon and water, which both play important roles in sexual energy. Many yoga asanas can open up this area, such as Goddess pose (deviasana), and you'll find essential oils of orange, sandalwood, or ylang-ylang help to awaken the powerful force of desire within you. This chakra's corresponding mantra sound is vam.

Another fantastic way to open your sacral chakra is through dance. If you take a minute right now to make circles with your hips, you'll start to feel the energy in this area shift straight away. No need to sign up for an official class, or even brave a crowded club on a Saturday night--crank up some music and dance in your bedroom. It might be best to do this in the privacy of your own home because you'll need to dismiss your inhibitions to get the most healing energy out of this practice.

Finally- this may seem obvious, but it can't be stressed enough--drink plenty of water. A dehydrated empath is likely to feel stagnant and stiff. You can hydrate this chakra by drinking water and consuming naturally orange foods, like tangerines or melons. It probably won't surprise you to learn that regular bathing can have a positive impact on your sexual energy, as well.

Solar Plexus Healing

Empaths typically have trouble keeping this chakra balanced, since we process so many more emotions here than the average person. You may want to seek guidance from a practitioner of Reiki or other healing arts while working to restore energetic balance here.

Consider adding more yellow squash and chamomile tea to your diet. An empath with an imbalanced solar plexus needs a boost of both confidence and calm. The squash is a solid complex carbohydrate to give you strong and sustainable energy during the day, while the tea will help to promote rest at night.

Boat pose (navasana) is great for activating or balancing the solar plexus chakra. If you feel this chakra is blocked, especially by emotional energy that you are ready to let go of, yoga twists of all kinds can be wonderfully healing. Think of your stomach like a rag oversaturated with liquid emotion; twisting and squeezing helps to purge the excess moisture, leaving only as much as the rag can comfortably hold. Though ultimately beneficial, yoga twists can be very challenging and uncomfortable for empaths, especially those suffering from emotional overload. Remember to take it slow to avoid injury, and breathe deeply throughout every step of your practice.

Empaths often feel pulled in a thousand different directions at once. We must remember that if we are pulled in too many different directions, we ultimately remain stationary. Choose to empower yourself. Pick one direction and take a step forward.

Make sure you are choosing forward momentum, and not fleeing from whatever is behind you. Your solar plexus chakra can differentiate between these two types of motion.

Heart Healing

This chakra's resonant color is green, so when the heart feels closed off or blocked, attract energy back towards it by incorporating more green into your wardrobe, diet, and home decor. Wear or carry green healing stones, like jade or green aventurine; eat green vegetables; bring some green plants into your home.

Gratitude is one of the simplest practices that can reverse the flow of energy in your heart chakra. It helps you to transform negativity into positive energy. You can express your gratitude through meditative thoughts, written manifestations, or verbal affirmations.

You may also wish to incorporate affirmations of self-love and universal love in your yoga and meditation practices.

Camel pose (ustrasana) is a perfect position to open up your heart chakra.

Throat Healing

Sing a song. Don't worry about the sound of your voice; instead, focus on your breath, making sure that the root power of your vocal projection is in your diaphragm, rather than your chest or throat. When song stems from the membrane, it is easy to avoid vocal strain, and you will feel the sonic vibrations of each note resonating throughout your body. If you can let go of self-consciousness, this sensation can be incredibly soothing and therapeutic. Experiment with different melodies; try singing or tantric chant with your body posed in different positions, as though attempting to scratch a sonic itch that's hard to reach. You can also try singing in different physical spaces; the size and shape of rooms, the height of ceilings, and flooring materials can all impact sonic vibrations, amplifying or absorbing their energy. This exercise can help you to stay mindful of the fact that effective communication is not just a matter of precise language and having the confidence to speak; context is also an integral part of the equation.

You may also want to take a break from technology and media for a few hours, even a full day if you're able. We constantly strain our necks and shoulders to use computers and mobile phones; we also tend to push our jaw bones forward when we are anxious, which strains the same muscle group. You can release tension from this area by taking many technology breaks and staying mindful of your posture throughout the day.

Fish pose (matsyana) is an ideal yoga pose to open the throat chakra. Lapis lazuli is the gemstone most commonly used to balance this area and enhance confidence in expression. Say confidence is not your problem, but you find yourself frequently misunderstood, with your words always lost in translation; in this case, opt for a transparent blue healing stone, like aquamarine or topaz. Meditate on truth, authenticity, and the nature of expression.

Third Eye Healing

An empath may wish to enhance the energy flow to the third eye to find greater clarity, or they might want to decrease the energy flow to this area if their empathic abilities are hyperactive.

Meditation can channel energy to the third eye. Grounding is an easy way to pull energy from an overactive third eye, redirecting the energy towards the three lowest chakras. Adequate, good quality sleep can be immensely helpful in balancing this chakra, whether it is overstimulated or lacking energy. You can also tailor your diet to promote healthy function in the pineal gland.

Both the third eye and crown chakras can benefit from scalp and face massages since these areas are typically overlooked in massage therapy. Be sure to focus some attention on the ears, temples, and forehead. Dolphin (makarasana) and child's pose (balasana) are excellent ways to channel energy to the third eye during your yoga practice.

As an empath, you can benefit from attending faith-based services, whether or not you are a believer. You'll be able to pick up on the energetic vibrations of other attendees and use them as a sort of short cut to third eye awakening. It won't be possible if you do not hold respect in your heart for everyone involved in the service, or if you bear a general sense of skepticism towards their faith. Keep your mind and heart open, and remember you have come to learn, not to judge.

Crown Healing

The crown chakra is spiritual, and since every individual maintains a unique relationship to the divine, there is no step-by-step guide to healing or balancing this chakra. Find a spiritual practice or journey that resonates with you, and remain open to guidance along the way. You'll have to rely on a firm foundation built by your other lower chakras, and trust your sensory perceptions to steer you towards the rituals that will serve you best. You might create an altar in a private area of your home, filled with crystals, natural materials like bone and petrified wood, candles or energy grids. You can try prayer, acupressure, or qigong to expand your spiritual perspective.

Meditation, again, is an invaluable skill for anyone seeking to enhance spirituality through the crown. The mantra sound "om" is used to channel energy to both the crown and the third eye in meditation or yoga practice. You can use lotus pose (padmasana) or plow pose (halasana) to activate the crown specifically.

Listen to the universe. Keep your eyes open and on the lookout for synchronicities. Even if you don't suspect yourself to be a precognitive empath, it may be helpful to start a dream journal or meditative journal and see if you can note any thought patterns that might be coming to you from a divine energy source rather than earthly, material stimulus.

Aromatherapy

Essential oils, incense, and scented candles have been used for thousands of years in metaphysical healing. You can incorporate them into meditation and yoga practices, reiki, or chakra healing sessions. To amplify self-love, you can use your favorite scents for a luxurious bath. Some essential oil blends can promote improved digestion, tension relief, and better quality sleep. You can also practice mindfulness by dabbing a drop of your favorite oil at the center of your upper lip, just below the nose, to help you stay conscious of your breathing patterns throughout the day. Keep in mind that you'll want to dilute most essential oils in a carrier oil before applying them directly to your skin.

There are many varied opinions about which essential oils are most useful for certain healing practices. In chakra healing, for instance, different oils and scents are recommended to resonate with each energy center in the body, yet not all healers agree on the specifics. Ultimately, so long as the aroma in question is natural (not synthetic) and pleasant for you to savor, you cannot go wrong with essential oils. Use them sparingly, as scents can often intensify under friction or heat, and start a log to keep note of which blends you find most effective.

Smudging

Smudging is an ancient Native American tradition that you can easily use to cleanse your living space, crystals, and even your chakras. It is a ritual burning of sacred herbs, using the smoke to wash a body, object or area of all blockages and negative energies.

Sage is the most commonly used herb in smudging, but there are plenty of other aromas to use if you're not fond of its scent. People also smudge with cedar, lavender, nag champa, copal, sweetgrass, mugwort, frankincense, and palo santo.

Experiment with a few different herbs; breathe in deeply and take note of how your body responds to the aromas. If you don't enjoy a particular scent, take note and stop burning it. That may be a sign that this herb is not serving your energetic needs, and another type of plant is needed for this cleansing.

Crystal Healing

There are hundreds of varieties of crystals, each with unique metaphysical properties and uses. Here, you'll find just a handful of the types that are most commonly used by empaths for cleansing, recharging, and healing.

It's a good idea to read up on your crystals before building a collection and use them mindfully. Crystals are more than just beautiful decorations; they store energetic charge, and they can become polluted with negative energies if they are poorly cared for. Wear your crystals, carry them with you, keep them close during meditation or yoga practice, and use them to decorate your haven space--but be selective. Using all your crystals, or too many different kinds at once, can weaken their net energy and render some of them powerless. Some crystals are like battery chargers for other crystals, cleansing and restoring their energy, while others are porous and delicate, absorbing energy from everything around them.

Your crystals will need to be regularly cleaned. You can do this in some different ways; smudging, as explained above, is one easy way to remove the negative charge and other forms of energy pollution from your healing stones. Moonlight is also a favorite cleansing agent, with best results found under the glow of a full moon. Some empaths bury their crystals underground for approximately twenty-four hours a few times a month to keep them cleansed and grounded. Sunlight, rainwater, spring water, and salt water can also be used to cleanse certain crystals, but use these methods with caution! Bright sunlight can lighten or discolor some gems, and porous stones can be easily damaged by water or scratched by salt.

Amethyst

Amethyst is a very popular and easily accessible stone that all empaths can benefit. You can use the stones in interior decor and chakra cleansing, or wear them as jewelry. Their beautiful light purple hue is great for accessorizing, and they make fantastic gifts for anyone in emotionally challenging situations.

Amethysts help to enhance intuition and promote mental clarity. These are ideal for anyone who wants to deepen their understanding of a dilemma or get more in touch with their empathic abilities.

Hematite

Hematite is a shiny, metallic dark grey stone with a highly reflective surface when polished. This iron-rich, semi-precious gemstone is excellent for accessorizing in jewelry or interior decoration, and it is a must-have for empaths.

Hematite can be great for protecting your boundaries and repelling energy vampires. Think of it as a reflective shield, using the "I am rubber, you are glue" defense against those who seek to deplete your energy reserves. It is also very useful at neutralizing anxiety.

Lepidolite

This crystal can sometimes look very similar to amethyst but is also often boasts more red, pink, or grey tones. It's a lithium bearing mineral that soothes and dissolves anxieties while promoting inner peace, so it's a natural choice for an empath. It also fits wonderfully into any crystal collection, because lepidolite functions like a crystal battery and amplifier, adding a strengthening power boost to any other stone you pair it with. It's also suitable for enhancing emotional intimacy with your loved ones, encouraging deep relaxation and restful sleep.

Carnelian

This bright red-orange stone is like a little piece of the sun that you can carry with you wherever you go, offering light, warmth, and energy. It is a physical healing stone, as it stimulates metabolic activity and blood flow. It also excellent for emotional healing, fueling a sense of empowerment, courage, and capability. It's wonderful to keep close if you are training for a significant challenge, like running a marathon, or when you are recovering from emotional trauma and abuse. When the empath feels depleted, carnelian will help them to feel reinvigorated and ready to move forward again.

Labradorite

This multicolored stone is a wonderful tool for creative types who need emotional stability and balance to pursue their goals, but also need the energy to stay motivated. It keeps the imagination active and sharpens intuition, while simultaneously promoting calm and removing anxieties. Labradorite is seen as a stone of transformation and can help you to achieve your goals or reach your higher purpose. It is also believed to be a good luck stone, assisting the users in avoiding misfortune.

Fluorite

This beautiful multicolored stone often includes a rainbow of pinks, purples, greens, blues, and whites. It is an excellent stone to balance the third eye chakra; it promotes a sense of calm, lifts and dissolves mental or emotional fog, drives spiritual awakening, and reminds us of the big picture or our divine purpose. Meditate with this gemstone if you are feeling lost or in need of guidance.

Rose Quartz

This beautiful light pink stone is relatively common and inexpensive, but it has a lot of metaphysical value. Quartz of any kind is great for grounding, but rose quartz, in particular, can help to solidify our sense of being unconditionally loved by others, and by the universe as a whole. It is an important thing for the empath to be reminded of, as most highly sensitive people have been repeatedly hurt in their past relationships.

Rose quartz is a powerful healing stone to use with the heart chakra, restoring balance and faith. It is also a natural go-to power stone for empaths who do not suffer from heartache or love troubles, because of its calming, soothing effects. It radiates enough unconditional love to keep us feeling emotionally steady and protected in crowded or chaotic environments, so it is great to carry in a pocket or wear as jewelry.

Magnetite

Magnetite is another powerful stone for grounding. It is naturally magnetic, and thus especially useful for balancing out the polarities of your energy field. Use magnetite in meditation or chakra healing whenever you are feeling is conflicted internally, or stuck in an emotional bind. It is also wonderful to keep present whenever you meet with other empaths or metaphysical healers because it helps both empaths to avoid taking on too much energy from the other, which can occasionally cause psychic overload. Its magnetic essence helps both empaths to keep their own emotions and energies reigned in and close to themselves, preventing leakage.

Apache Gold

This gorgeous black and gold stone is also sometimes called "Healer's gold," though it doesn't appear to have as much of a beneficial impact on physical health as it does on emotional restoration. This stone is a must-have for anyone who struggles with boundaries (and let's be honest, that group includes all empaths, no matter how advanced or empowered they may be). It helps to strengthen the resolve of your boundaries, as well as communicate your needs. It also absorbs negativity. Remember, stones that absorb negativity are doing something different than stones which deflect or dissolve it; apache gold absorbs negative energy, so it will need to be regularly cleaned. Otherwise, it will reintroduce negativity to your energy field every time you use it.

Malachite

This rich dark green stone is precious to empaths because it can dissolve and flush away emotional clogs. Used regularly, it will enhance your ability to identify and promptly release emotions correctly. Think of it as a metaphysical chiropractor, finding the hidden kinks in your emotional body, unraveling knots of tension, and sending you off a little lighter and taller than you were beforehand.

Malachite is also quite useful at negative cleansing energies from technology, so it's wise to keep this stone close at hand by the computer or tv, in kitchens with lots of appliances, or even in rooms with too much fluorescent lighting. You might want to invest in a malachite charm or key ring to keep close to your mobile phone at all times. This stone is only useful in its polished form, so avoid rough malachite, and stick to dry cleansing methods--no spring or sea water.

Black Tourmaline

This stone is a necessity for geomantic empaths. It has a very strong connection to the earth and can channel unwelcome energies back into the earth to be transformed and reborn. It also has immensely powerful protective abilities and is therefore quite useful for other empath types. It deflects and repels negativity, so it can help you to build an effective energy shield. Jet black, shiny, and durable, this is a great stone to carry or wear daily, especially when you know you'll be in contact with domineering or persuasive personalities. It can be a wonderful tool for empaths who suspect they may be stuck in a relationship with a narcissist or other empathy-deficient type, as it helps to prevent the dominant personality from projecting shame onto the empath; this encourages the narcissist to transform by interrupting their primary self-defensive response pattern and forcing them to explore other options.

Use with caution--this is an extremely powerful stone, and its impact on unhealthy relationships can be intense and unpredictable. It may be a catalyst for the ending of relationships that you are still sentimentally attached to, even though they are no longer serving you. When you invite this stone into your life, be prepared for significant, cataclysmic change.

Herkimer Diamonds and Clear Quartz

These two stones do have some different metaphysical properties, but one thing they have in common is their ability to heighten psychic awareness. These are both wonderful to use when you wish to improve your empathic skills or advance to a higher level of sensitive clarity. They're recommended for those who possess geomantic, claircognizant or precognitive empathy and wish to understand better the messages they receive.

These stones can deepen psychic attunement when used on their own, but they are also powerful amplifiers of the metaphysical properties in other crystals, so be careful what you pair them with, and cleanse these stones often.

Citrine, Obsidian, and Blue Lace Agate

Each of these stones is unique and possesses plenty of other beneficial metaphysical properties--but they are particularly useful for empaths who suffer from digestive disorders. These stones all promote healing of the gastrointestinal tract by purging negativity and unaddressed emotional blockages, which are often so deeply buried that we are not even conscious of them. Citrine especially can work as a powerful shield for the solar plexus chakra. Again, be sure to cleanse these stones thoroughly and frequently, lest they become charged with powerful negative energies.

8

Staying Light

It's beautiful to incorporate metaphysical healing into your self-care routine, but empaths must also develop real-world strategies to manage interpersonal relationships. In this chapter, we'll discuss how empaths can maintain positive energy and avoid taking on the burden of other people's emotional weight through behavioral change.

Be Selective

All humans crave love and emotional closeness, whether we are comfortable with intimacy or not. This desire is hard-wired in our brains, and as we grow up, society works to reinforce the idea that popularity is a useful metric by which to measure all forms of human success. We come to believe that people who are well-liked, with lots of friends and loved ones, are more virtuous people; that they are happier, healthier, have more successful careers, and lead more comfortable lives than those who have smaller social circles or spend a great deal of time alone.

Unfortunately, an empath who spends a great deal of time or energy chasing popularity might as well go ahead and shoot themselves in the foot, because this path holds very little promise for them. Popularity can often be a mirage--it looks like a miraculous oasis from a distance, but up close, it is rarely as pleasant as it seems. Especially for an empath, who takes on the emotions of those around them, popularity can feel like a prison. Popular people are often surrounded by various types of insecurity, self-hatred, narcissism, desperation, materialism, shallow value structures, and cognitive dissonance. In the face of popularity, people are often dishonest to others and themselves. Some will even adopt a cut-throat attitude. It is a disastrous emotional environment for an empath to land themselves in.

As hard as it may be to give up on the comforts that popularity promises, empaths must learn to be highly selective about the kind of company, they keep, as well as how much time and energy they spend around other people. All humans with typical ranges of empathetic sensitivity are influenced by the behaviors of the people they spend the most time with, subtly tailoring ourselves to navigate the preferences of those we love. But empaths take this habit a step further. Their surroundings don't merely influence them; they start to *become* their friends and family members after long periods of exposure to them, especially if the empath is untrained.

An easy place to start purging negativity from your life is through your social circle. Take a mental inventory of everyone you've spent a significant amount of time with this month, or this year if your memory allows it. Do you feel at peace with the activities and people you gave your time? Did you encounter any unpleasant or uncomfortable experiences that you feel, in retrospect, could have been avoided? And most importantly, how would you feel if this was the shape of your future, too? If you spent the rest of your life with these people, doing these same activities? This question may be difficult to answer honestly at first, especially if it alerts you to the fact that your values aren't entirely aligned with the values of your loved ones.

This exercise can also be a wake-up call for empaths who are living more for other people than they are for themselves. If you are primarily dissatisfied with the memories you've just reviewed, then you'll need to get into the habit of frequently asking yourself: "Why am I doing this?" If the answer is usually about needing to please other people or avoid angering them, or even a fear of adverse judgment from others, that's something to take note of and work to change.

Empaths thrive in authenticity. It may not sound as glamorous as sheer popularity, but having a handful of deep, authentic friendships will ultimately serve to make you much happier in the long run. Aim to gather a circle of friends that you feel you can be entirely honest with, even about your insecurities. You'll also find it much easier to manage your fluctuating energy levels with a supportive group of friends who understand your need for occasional solitude and don't employ peer pressure tactics to influence your behaviors.

You may realize some people in your life have brought you more emotional pain than joy. Ending relationships is always painful for empaths, even if they know it's ultimately for the best--but be mindful of the fact that there is no need for an official break up or spectacular display. You can merely minimize your exposure to negative people and allow your friendships to fade away over time gradually. If the negative person is uncooperative with your efforts to distance yourself, then you may need to explicitly tell them that you no longer wish to invest energy into the relationship, but there is no need to argue with them or insult them. They'll be more likely to respect your wishes if you claim the issue is your own, not their fault.

Lastly, remember that you do not owe anyone your friendship or even your attention, regardless of how long you've known them or how intricately they are woven into the rest of your social circle. Your emotional body may send you conflicting signals since it is used to being affected by external stimulus without warning or consent. But you do get to choose which emotional energies you will or will not engage with. All you need to do is get comfortable with setting boundaries.

The Basics of Boundaries

Boundary work is a necessity for all empaths. Since we are so deeply attuned to the emotions of other people, we must be distinctly conscious of where our feelings, desires, and emotional needs end and where those belonging to other people begin.

Imagine you live in an environmental utopia, where it is always pleasantly warm and dry, without rain or violent wind storms. You live in this place with a small harmonious community--say, for example, that ten other people are living here. Perhaps two or three of these people are your family and close friends; one might be your lover or closest companion; the rest are either mild acquaintances or people you're not at all fond of.

Imagine, now, that every person in this community has their own living space, their food and water supply, and their own collection of possessions for comfort and entertainment. But none of the homes has any walls. Ask yourself: without physical barriers to mark the borders between individuals, how would you go about establishing and protecting your personal space? How might you feel about sharing your resources, knowing everyone else has their supply of food and water, too? How comfortable would you feel in wandering into another person's living space without an invitation? If a family member of a friend decided to enter your space without warning, helping themselves to your resources, how might you react? Would you be equally welcoming to them if they came over happy, or sad, or angry, or even sleepy? And would you react differently if it were, instead, one of the people you don't like who came around and started eating all of your food?

You might be chuckling to yourself right now, thinking: "Obviously, if it bothered me, I would tell them to leave, and instruct them to ask my permission the next time they want to enter my space." If that is your reaction, then you may already have a pretty firm understanding of healthy boundaries without even being conscious of it. Unfortunately, the concept of clearly communicating your limits, or verbally establishing boundaries, isn't obvious to everyone. A lot of us empaths especially struggle even to recognize our own needs, let alone articulate them to others in an effective way. We sometimes expect other people to anticipate our boundaries without any signal or communication from us, which can lead to unnecessary disappointment and conflict. And to make matters even more confusing, loads of apparently high-functioning adults in this world don't have any personal boundaries at all, nor do they understand that they ought to respect the boundaries of others. These people have a destabilizing effect on boundary culture as a whole because they put other people in the position of having to explain, justify, or validate their limits by comparison. They often project an attitude that says: "I don't mind it when people invade my privacy, so if you're bothered by invasions of your personal space, that must mean there is something wrong with you."

Love stories and tales of close companionship in popular culture often model extremely unhealthy relationships for us; wherein there are no boundaries at all, overly rigid boundaries, or flimsy boundaries that are repeatedly ignored in the name of grand romantic gestures. The lessons we learn from these stories are misleading, teaching us that compatible friends or lovers ought to be able to read our minds, even through misleading signals, and that explicitly asking for our needs to be met is uncool or unattractive. Sadly, modern technology has served to make the maintenance of healthy boundaries even more difficult in recent times. The demands of social media applications are overshadowing the human need for occasional privacy, solitude, and rest. Many people now feel they are expected to be available and on-call for work and social obligations twenty-four hours a day, seven days a week, with an unfailing gregarious disposition, and camera-ready throughout every second of their lives.

Studies have shown that most of us create social media posts to overcompensate for our insecurities. We might post a photo that portrays us as happy and joyous when we are unfortunate or writes a post that explains how busy we are when in actuality, we are bored and lonely. These applications allow us to project a tailored image of the lives we wish we were leading, without ever addressing or inspiring the change we need to improve our overall satisfaction in the real world. So through social media, we are all making a systematic practice of saying the opposite of what we mean, projecting dishonesty and mixed messages, and investing energy into stagnation rather than growth. If you know anything about ritual manifestation, then you probably already realize what a dangerous practice this is.

Aside from the fact that this kind of projection can disrupt your connection to higher realms, it will likely also have a corrupting influence on the boundaries in your relationships. If you are deeply entrenched in social media use and feel frequently drained, anxious, overwhelmed, or inadequate, do yourself a favor and take a hiatus to reconnect with your unplugged self. Think about your boundaries in the physical world; how much time do you like to spend alone, versus in the company of others? How often do you invite others into your personal space? Do you enjoy being stared at in the real world? When you walk down the street or go shopping for groceries, how much do you allow the opinions of strangers to influence your feelings about yourself?

Your standards for the real world and the virtual world of social media should be primarily aligned. If you don't enjoy small talk with strangers in real life, then there's no reason why you should force yourself to endure the same on a social media platform. Through a web interface, other people will often react harshly to anything they perceive as rejection, so be prepared for plenty of people to question, disregard, or even berate your boundaries. Remember that you do not owe anyone an explanation of why your limits are what they are.

If you understand the need to ask for consent before making a sexual advance on another person, then you understand boundaries. Just as every person has different limits and preferences in the bedroom, we all have different boundaries in life, depending on our level of comfort with intimacy and other factors, like cultural or socio-economic background. Respecting someone's boundaries essentially means that in all parts of life outside the bedroom, you ask for consent rather than making assumptions about their limits, and you are ready to pull back whenever they say "no." When you define your boundaries, you are essentially making a contract with yourself, determining what kinds of treatment you will or will not tolerate from others, and promising to follow through with established consequences if people in your life cannot respect these boundaries. Your boundaries can be flexible; you may decide that they need to be moved in response to unusual circumstances, or your boundaries may fall in different places with different people in your life. For example, one of my boundaries is that I need complete privacy in the bathroom; no one--not even my partner--is welcome to enter the bathroom if I've closed the door behind me. But this boundary can be flexible if I am sick, or my partner is, and one of us needs assistance in the bathroom. I can bend this rule with my partner, but I keep this boundary rigid with friends and acquaintances.

Boundaries can be difficult to establish if you haven't gotten into the practice early in life. But it is never too late to start improving your relationships with clear communication and boundary work. This work doesn't have to be an official meeting, nor does it require two people to agree on a set of boundaries. You must determine your boundaries for yourself, and decide on your terms how you will apply them. People may not respect your limits, but if they don't, it's up to you to either communicate your boundaries more clearly or stop giving this person the opportunity to cross them.

Empaths tend to think outwardly, meaning we are more focused on other people than we are on ourselves. That being the case, many of us have trouble putting boundary work into practice initially, as we are stuck in a mindset that believes boundaries need to held up by the people on both sides of them. This is not the case, and so it may be helpful to stop envisioning boundaries as walls or barriers. Instead, think of your limits as represented by your physical body. Your skin serves to separate what is inside of you from everything else in the world, holding in everything essential and allowing that which isn't helping you to be eliminated. Your skin doesn't require cooperation from any other person or exterior force to continue holding your life essence in or to keep exterior elements, like rain, out. Your body can choose to be flexible about its boundaries, opening the mouth to let nourishment in, or purging infection through a ruptured cyst. Most importantly, it doesn't require permission or validation from any exterior source to continue doing its work.

Imagine yourself as a tightrope walker in a busy, hectic circus. You are high above the crowd, trying to get from point A to point B without falling--that is your only goal. Meanwhile, all around you, ahead, behind, and below, people are screaming, waving, watching. Other circus performers beneath you are running, dancing, leaping, spitting fire. There are moving spotlights above you, glaring, and bright camera flashes going off all around, unpredictably.

You can't allow any of those distractions to startle you or throw you off-balance. To walk across the room, you must focus exclusively on your balance.

That is an excellent analogy for the empath because this is necessarily what you have to do every day to take care of your own needs and avoid the pitfalls of emotional energy pollution. Can you imagine how much harder this task would be for a circus performer who couldn't see or feel the tightrope but had to get across the room by walking on blind faith? That's what it's like for an empath to try and survive without a clearly defined set of boundaries and personal goals. If you don't know the trajectory of your tightrope like the back of your hand, then you're just scrambling forward, hoping to float instead of falling, and that situation isn't likely to end well.

What is an Energy Vampire?

Also frequently called the "psychic vampire," the energy vampire is a person who has grown intolerant of their own naturally uncomfortable emotions, such as guilt, shame, confusion or anxiety, and so they have developed the habit of projecting those emotions onto others, passing them on as in a game of hot potato. Meanwhile, the energy vampire leeches positivity from others for their own needs and does not return any positive energy to those they've drained in the process. They are sometimes (but not always) narcissistic or otherwise empathy-deficient, and usually, seem oblivious to the fact that their emotional needs are exhausting the people around them. And they love empaths, so there's a perfect chance you already know a few of these people.

This form of vampirism isn't a fixed state. It's relatively common for people to go through phases of vampiric behavior when their emotional energy field has been injured, after a traumatic experience, for instance, or following an ugly break up. We all know what this familiar dynamic looks like: if your friend tells you they've been dealt a rough hand this week and could use some support, you invite them over, feed them comfort food, and let them express all the negative feelings they've been holding inside.

You offer a shoulder to cry on, a few encouraging words, maybe even a back rub or a drink. You don't expect your friend to ask many questions about your life at this point, but you can be reasonably sure that they'll express gratitude for your support and do their very best to reciprocate when their energy is balanced again.

But if you know someone who seems to expect this sort of emotional pampering from you, yet never seems genuinely interested in sending some of that restorative energy back your way, it's likely that you've got a real psychic vampire on your hands. You may be better off ending the relationship; if you can't, you'll want to minimize your exposure to this person until they've done some serious emotional growth.

A lot of empaths may have close friendships with energy vampires, only to gradually grow apart or even definitively cut off the connection over a disagreement. Energy vampires are drawn to empaths, because we often mirror their emotional responses immediately and to a similar degree, which gives them a feeling of catharsis.

Most narcissists are energy vampires, but not all energy vampires have a narcissistic personality disorder. Both types have a tendency to presume their personal needs or feelings are more important than those of other people, but the energy vampire might be entirely unaware of the impact of their behavior, and if it is brought to their attention, they may feel genuinely remorseful and ashamed of their actions. Narcissists would instead cling to the idea that they are better than those they've hurt, and that the pain they've caused is therefore justifiable.

If you know an energy vampire and suspect that they honestly have good intentions buried somewhere underneath all that volatile emotional projection, then you might want to try and steer them towards self-awareness--but be sure to proceed with caution! This person may be what some call a "covert narcissist," rejecting common markers of narcissistic behavior like flashy clothing and braggadocious claims, and instead relying on self-pity for attention. Your attempt to help them may be turned around into another song and dance focused primarily on sympathy and wallowing, rather than healing and growth.

Furthermore, energy vampires are used to leaning on others when they ought to be standing on their legs, so you can't heal this vicious cycle by continuing it. Don't do the healing work for them. You can't have a revelation of self-awareness on someone else's behalf.

An energy vampire may tend to treat you like a human version of a web-based search engine, asking you for information and guidance that they could easily find on their own if they would try to be self-sufficient. They also often have conflicted relationships with their actual parents, and thus spend much of their adult lives thrusting friends, lovers, and even co-workers into parental roles, whether those roles are wanted or not. These habits mean that even an energy vampire with an earnest desire to change may end up treating you like it's your job to fix them without expecting payment or reciprocation, especially if you're the one to open their eyes to the problem.

Don't indulge this impulse. A child never learns to stand on their own two feet until the parent stops cradling, let's go and allows them to flail around on the floor for a while. It can be painful for an empath to watch the flailing, but it is a necessary part of the growth process. Try sitting on your hands if you can't resist the urge to help. You'll want to save your healing energy for someone ready to receive and nurture it, rather than a vampire who will treat it like a disposable, bottomless resource. Even with good intentions, an energy vampire is liable to drink from your well until it has run completely dry, at which point they will promptly turn their backs to you and go searching for another well. If you stop this cycle in its tracks by cutting them off from your healing energy, the vampire is much more likely to look within themselves to find their energy source, rather than continue relying on external supply.

It's also important to remember that you can never force an awakening, reckoning, or any form of growth upon anyone. It's often a waste of an empath's time and energy to take on the role of a mentor or recovery coach because we are so likely to meet people more than halfway, making the healing process easier for them than it is meant to be an absorbing the split difference ourselves. Be wary of any "reformed" energy vampire who frequently reminds you that they could not have come this far without your guidance. If a person truly wishes to grow and change, they will find a way to take the first few steps of that journey with or without your help. Don't ever let yourself become the linchpin in someone else's recovery process, because you'll find they can just as quickly turn around and blame you for all of their failures and missteps, too.

How to create an energy shield

First, be aware that energy shields cannot be fueled by thought and intention alone. To keep your guard strong, you'll need a foundation of consistent self-care through proper rest, nutrition, physical activity, meditative practice, avoidance of toxic interactions, and the incorporation of an authentic lifestyle. Think of your energy shield as a set of turrets atop the temple that is your emotional self. The walls and foundation of the temple have to be solidly built and well-maintained to support the weight of their defense system.

You can use a physical talisman or crystal to activate your shield or to store energetic charge for it. Most empaths practice creating the shield without props, though, so that they can enable it at the drop of a hat, under any set of circumstances.

Activating your shield is primarily a visualization technique. First, envision your aura, a halo of light surrounding your entire body and spiritual essence. It may have a color, or it may be pure divine light. Next, you'll need to determine what kind of shield you want to cast. Is your primary goal to avoid drama and stay focused on your goals? Or to preserve personal energy levels? Perhaps you want to absorb love but deflect negativity. Visualize each of these forces as a physical entity, and then imagine yourself forging a shield of light, buzzing with energetic charge, to suit your needs.

Many metaphysical healers and guides have their methods for casting energetic shields. Ask your yoga teachers, reiki masters, spiritual guides and fellow empaths if they have any advice for personalizing this practice or honing your technique.

Letting go of expectations

Empaths feel genuinely, and it can be challenging for us to understand how their emotions don't drive other people. Sometimes, we expect other people to feel compelled, as we do, to do the right thing, express compassion to those in need, stifle the energy supplies of people with malicious intent, foster deep connections, and seek out higher truths. We are often in awe of people who can let things go smoothly; we may fear this behavior in other people, especially when they can quickly let go of things or people that we believe they ought to feel a sentimental attachment.

It may sound cynical, but learning to lower your expectations of other people can be incredibly freeing for empaths. In truth, many people you meet simply won't express any interest in the things that matter most to you. Deep levels of empathy are terrifying for some people, and entirely inaccessible for others still. Throughout your life, you will encounter a significant number of people who never practice reciprocity or gratitude, and never pay any mind to their emotional bodies. If you expect them to do so, you will feel disappointment. If you expect nothing, what you will feel instead is either an impulse to ask explicitly for the attention you need, or an ability to accept things as they are, and be at peace with them.

9

Finding Empathic Joy

When you purge negative energy from your life, you'll want to fill the void created by that negativity with sources of sheer joy and positivity. You may feel the impulse to turn to vices or addictions at this time, but below you'll find healthier practices to invest in. Choosing these things over alcohol, adrenaline rushes, or sexual gratification will pay off in the long run, as they will nourish positivity inside you, rather than draining your energy or throwing your ego into a state of imbalance.

Plants and Nature

Even if you are not a plant empath, nurturing seeds to growth can help restore your faith in your capabilities, as well as in the magic of the universe.

Spending time in nature can help to foster spiritual awakening, restore emotional balance, and cleanse emotional contagion from your energy field. It is also an effective cure for loneliness, reminding us that walls are human constructions, and without them, none of us is ever truly alone.

Animals and Children

Empaths can sometimes get a natural high from spending time with animals or young children. These spirits resonate with ours in a way that many other adults cannot, since they rely so heavily on empathic knowledge to navigate their way through life. They can make us laugh, remind us to release our inhibitions, and show us that we are unconditionally loved.

Creative Expressions

Without expression, an empath can quickly turn into an emotional powder keg. Whether creativity is your life's great passion, or you struggle to find a form of artistic expression that feels comfortable for you, your empathic energy can always benefit from trying to channel a message through an artistic medium.

There is no right or wrong form of creativity to embrace, nor do you need to exhibit any particular skill or talent to get a lot out of it. The goal is to enjoy the practice, or get some sense of catharsis from it--if you're lucky, you'll be able to kill those two birds with one stone. Try as many different forms of creative expression as you can, but if you need some guidance in deciding where to start, then knowing your empath type might help to steer you in a promising direction.

If you are a plant empath, you may want to consider acting. That might sound irrelevant, but gardening and staging a play utilize a lot of the same skills. The plant empath might enjoy this opportunity to express themselves to an audience without having to endure a lot of back and forth, exerting total control over their scene work. As in a garden, on stage, the actor works to plant the idea of a world or story within the audience and nurtures the concept until it grows fully realized. As in a garden, a thousand little energies need to work in perfect synchronization to achieve the desired effect; and ultimately, the result, though beautiful, is temporary. Acting is a form of art that lives.

If you are a physical empath, dance is a fairly obvious choice. Physical empaths run the risk of putting too much focus on the bodies of others, failing to attend to their own needs. Dancing will help the physical empath to stay grounded in their own body while releasing tensions and expressing emotion. Circus arts can also be therapeutic for the physical empath, as they aim to express the inner self through larger than life gestures. Many circus arts require an enormous focus on proprioception, which is the mental map you hold of your body's shape, size, placement, and movement when you have no access to a mirror or spatial place marker. Again, physical empaths can easily lose their sense of proprioception by channeling so much energy into understanding other people's bodies rather than their own. To test your proprioception, close your eyes and stretch your arms up over your head. You can wave them around or shake them out to release tension, but then, with your eyes still closed, try to find the tip of your nose with your pointer finger. If you missed the mark or hit yourself a little harder than you intended to, your proprioception needs some work. For a more challenging test, stand sideways by a mirror, close your eyes, and lift one leg until you feel that your thigh bone is about parallel to the floor. Now open your eyes and check your alignment in the mirror. How did you do? Proprioception can be enhanced through all kinds of physical activities, but yoga and dance are particularly useful because they focus on kinetic balance.

Geomantic empaths might find sculpture, woodwork, or stone carving to be both meditative and a dominant form of creative expression. Working with these mediums requires both force and a gentle touch, as the materials can sometimes be fickle, stubborn and delicate. They may also be drawn to metalsmithing or jewelry design with healing crystals and precious gemstones, which carry incredible amounts of stored energy from the earth and universe. Did you know, for example, that all of the gold on this planet fell to earth inside of meteorites over three billion years ago? Or that glassy, rare moldavite was formed in the heat of a sudden impact, and thus can be seen as a physical manifestation of a historical, cosmic event? Geomantic empaths are especially encouraged to use fire and heat to mold and shape precious metals or other materials, as this practice will help them to feel deeply connected to the same creative forces that shaped our universe billions of years ago.

Animal empaths are likely to enjoy singing or other forms of musical expression, as it makes use of many of the same non-verbal elements that are used to communicate with animals, while at the same time articulating some distinctly human concepts, such as the structured order of rhythm or harmony. Music speaks to universal emotions and is a powerful tool for the misunderstood to use when they need to feel heard and valued. It has been proven to be physiologically and psychologically beneficial for humans to listen, and even more so to perform in chorus with others. In recent years, several scientific fields have experimented with the effect music has on animals, finding that some species like birds and cows can appreciate human musicality. Cows produce more milk if they are made to listen to relaxing tunes while grazing and milking. Some species like cats appear uninterested in human music, but songs that are written to suit their sonic range and preferred tempos better will catch their attention. Elephants are particularly musically inclined, able to play instruments that are specially designed to be played with the trunk, and sometimes able to hold a steady rhythm better than a human drummer could!

Emotional empaths, being the most common, will enjoy many different creative mediums, but painting, illustration, poetry and prose writing seem to resonate exceptionally well with this type. These forms of expression help to translate the intangible into a precise, well-defined, permanent medium, which allows the empath to release their internal emotions indeed.

Join a Group with a Unified Goal

Since empaths can pick up on so many energy levels, they may find their energy fields frequently disturbed by a sense of constant conflict. At any given moment, every person on this planet wants something, is working towards a goal of some kind, and whether these goals are large or small, they are often in conflict with one another. Tapping into this reality can be exhausting for empaths, or in severe cases, a catalyst for depression and feelings of hopelessness.

To combat these feelings, you may find it extremely useful to join a group that meets regularly to work towards a common goal. If the group is well managed and its members mostly have honest intentions, this type of harmonious atmosphere can help to restore your energy and faith in humanity. Joining a singing group or choir can be especially useful in achieving this goal. You might join a church or faith-based organization. Sports teams can be great, but if the sport is hyper-competitive or has a violent nature, it may not be very therapeutic for an empath. If the group is building something together without any need for internal competition, it will help you to feel powerful, valuable, and held up by the world, rather than lost in its aether or at odds with it.

Be careful of any group whose only goal is fundraising. Even if the cause is incredible, environments that are primarily focused on money are not ideal for empaths. Money is a physical representation of power, and we empaths don't enjoy taking power away from others, nor are we inclined to hoard more of it than we need at any given time. These environments are likely to awaken an anxious or stressed response inside of us, rather than bringing us joy. There is nothing wrong with fundraising or earning money honestly, but empaths are not naturally good with money, so our energies can be put to better use elsewhere.

Physical Manifestation

As an empath, you may suffer from mental or emotional overload. It can be overwhelming and exhausting to keep so many of your own emotions balanced inside you while warding off negative energies from external sources and allowing positive and neutral energies to flow through. To stay focused, present, and firm in your sense of self, you must adopt the practice of frequent physical manifestation. That is how you will regularly project your rich, complex inner world into the physical realm. It may be as simple as making a daily list of gratitudes, desires, or personal priorities; it might be a more abstract and creative form of manifestation, like painting the things you see in your head when you close your eyes, dancing to express feeling, songwriting, collage, or any form of expression that appeals to you. Some empaths prefer manifestation rituals that involve crystal healing, celestial alignment events, or prayer to divine deities.

It may take some experimentation and practice to find a manifestation ritual that works well for you, but if you work diligently towards this goal, you will eventually find yourself much more energized, balanced, and emotionally stable. Think of your mind as a kitchen counter; to cook anything efficiently, you need enough clear and clean space, your ingredients easily at hand, and a plan for how you'll chop, mix, season or heat them all. Physical manifestation is a way to clear all the unnecessary ingredients from the counter, lay out all the cookware you'll need close at hand, and highlight the relevant recipe. It's a way to set yourself up for success, so even the challenging parts of life feel easy to manage.

Forgiveness

Forgiveness is neither a word nor a concept to take lightly. Studies in both psychology and neuroscience have proven that it can have an impressive beneficial impact on both the person granting forgiveness and the person who is forgiven, reducing overall stress levels, lowering blood pressure and improving auto-immune function for both parties.

If you are an empath, there is a high probability that you have been deeply hurt in past relationships. You may find yourself struggling to move on, to stop caring, or to let go of angry feelings. That is natural, especially if the person (or people) who caused you pain has not done anything to express remorse. Still, forgiveness isn't about justice (which might be why some empaths struggle with the concept since we tend to value fairness very highly); forgiveness is about releasing negative energy, and making space for joy. Don't ask yourself if this person deserves your forgiveness--instead, ask yourself if you are ready to let go of the weight of your anger, pain, and hurt feelings. Ask yourself if you are prepared to move forward.

If you are honest with yourself, you might find that you are not yet ready to forgive. This is perfectly fine, so long as you are willing to work through your anger and learn from it. Don't let anger sit unattended inside of you, where it can grow roots. Anger is meant to be a motivator, inspiring you to grow and change. If you aren't ready to forgive, then it may mean that your passion needs to be more closely examined and analyzed for you to find a lesson within it.

When you are ready to forgive, you'll also feel inclined to invite more joy into your life. You can use a forgiveness ritual to mark the beginning of a new chapter in your life story, but you can also choose to close your eyes and radiate the energy of compassion. You do not necessarily have to be in contact with someone to forgive them; they do not need to be involved in the process at all. Forgiveness is about the forgiver, not the overlooked, and sometimes it's as simple as deciding not to dwell on the past for another minute, focusing all of your energy on the present instead.

LKM Daily Practice

LKM stands for loving-kindness meditation. It is a very simple ritual, and studies have shown that incorporating it into your daily meditative practice is, in essence, a way to warm up and stretch your brain's empathy muscles, keeping them in good shape, ready to handle whatever life throws at them.

This practice takes only a few minutes. Find a quiet and soothing place to sit and close your eyes. Send out love and genuine goodwill, systematically, in the following order: first, to your loved ones; secondly, to someone you're not on good terms with at the moment. Third, send loving thoughts to every soul on the planet that is plagued by suffering; lastly, turn that love back towards yourself, forgive yourself for your failures and missteps, and send yourself a kind thought or two, acknowledging that you are worthy of such kindness.

10

Finding Peace

Regardless of our empathic abilities or lack thereof, we all aim to fill our lives with as much joy as possible. Using the tools and strategies outlined in previous pages, the empath should find that their overall level of happiness generally increases. As it becomes easier to recognize and manage the different types of energies that surround them, it will also become more comfortable to be selective and make consistently positive choices.

Still, even for those who have mastered these skills and choose to focus all of their energy on positivity, constant and everlasting joy is an unrealistic goal to strive for. We all have our blind spots, vulnerabilities, and weaknesses. Sooner or later, the empowered empath will encounter a source of negativity that they cannot (or just do not wish to) ignore, compartmentalize, or remedy.

It is in those moments, where joy is not accessible, that the empath must learn to find a way to inner peace instead. Imagine, for example, that someone you love and deeply respect has passed away. It would be ludicrous for anyone, even an empowered empath, to expect to find their way to true joy during the funerary services, or at any point within the mourning period. Whatever your views on death and the possibility of an afterlife may be, a loss of this magnitude is always painful. If the empath wishes to attend a wake or funeral, they'll certainly need to prepare themselves for the experience, utilizing whatever strategies they need to avoid taking on pain of other mourners in the room. However, the empath who is focused exclusively on seeking joy may run the risk of ignoring their genuine feelings of pain, thereby distancing the self from emotions and feelings that belong to no one else. This is a dangerous practice for any empath to grow accustomed to, as it can be seductively pleasant at first; but much like the alcoholic who avoids the pain of a hangover by consistently consuming the hair of the dog that bit them, the empath will find that they can never outrun their own emotions, even if they aim to shut them out in the same way that they shut out the feelings of negative people.

. . .

Balance, ultimately, is a superior goal. An empath with a strong sense of inner balance can attend a funeral, commiserate with others, honor their sadness, and process feelings of grief without being consumed by them. Their balance allows them to recognize that sorrow is not an opposing force to happiness, but preferably that it is a functional part of joy; that without misery, we would never feel bliss, or perhaps anything at all.

Over time, the empath will learn that this state of equilibrium is indeed their most heightened state of being and the place where they will find their real self.

Embrace Discomfort

Here's a revolutionary idea that can take your yoga, tai chi, or mindfulness practice to the next level: discomfort is just an emotion. It isn't real. It isn't a threat, but it is a motivator.

Embracing discomfort isn't the same as numbing yourself to it. When you accept cognitive dissonance or moral injustices, you numb yourself to discomfort, embracing apathy and encouraging the distortion of the truth. When you allow yourself to experience discomfort without immediately reacting, however, you can learn to make empowered choices, overcome fears and anxieties, and reach towards emotional growth. For empaths, discomfort is often a sensation of uncertainty or anticipation of conflict. If you can learn to recognize the feeling without letting it trigger your fight or flight response, you can instead focus on taking productive action, making yourself the true master of your universe.

That is an enlightened position that very few humans take. If you can start to use your discomfort as a tool, rather than avoiding it at all costs, you may find yourself able to overcome challenges that leave others destroyed. Once you've mastered this technique, do your best to pay it forward to another empath.

Live an Authentic Life

One thing that can throw any empath off balance and block the pathway to inner peace is a lack of authenticity in your lifestyle. Empaths often carry lies or dishonesty inside for long periods, haunted by them, even allowing the memory of them to block their throat, heart, and solar plexus chakras. That being the case, it's best for empaths to avoid lying whenever possible--even white lies can cause disruptions in your energy field.

You can work towards this goal through both addition and elimination. For addition, make a point to invite positive energy flow into your life by aligning your career, personal relationships, eating habits and hobbies with your value system. For example, if you have come to realize that environmentalism is deeply important to you, then pursuing work in green planning would be a fantastic first step. You could also reach out to foster new friendships with people who are passionate about the same causes; you might alter your diet to favor organic, locally sourced produce, and make a heightened effort to buy from environmentally conscious companies.

For elimination, you'll want to start purging anything from your life that puts you in a position of moral conflict. If your job or social circle are not environmentally-conscious, you'll be under constant pressure to swallow your truth and project dishonesty, which will ultimately leave you feeling dissatisfied and ungrounded. Any relationship wherein you feel the need to lie to keep everyone happy is a bad relationship for you, and you should feel free to let go of it.

You'll also want to stop using your money to support brands whose values contradict your own, and give up any habits that have a negative impact on the things that matter most to you--for instance, if you love poetry, song, and other forms of vocal expression, it's may be time to quit smoking cigarettes once and for all. You might be pleasantly surprised to notice your physical body and spiritual energy shift in a tangible way once you release the cognitive dissonance you once held inside yourself. You'll feel lighter, taller, more dynamic, and more capable.

I'll include another reminder here to be careful with social media use. Sometimes, these applications can do a lot of good to bring people together and inject dynamic momentum into progressive movements--but most often, they are cesspools of inauthentic energy. Aim to use these platforms sparingly, if at all, and to post honestly and responsibly.

Choosing Humility and Respecting the Unknown

No matter how empowered one may become, and regardless of how well one has honed their empathic power, it is crucial to embrace humility keep the mind open to unexpected possibilities. The self-righteous empath who develops a hermetic view of the world, unwilling to entertain ideas that do not strongly resonate with their interior knowledge, is likely to be deeply discontented or anxious, and struggle with communication and loving relationships, as others will perceive them to be arrogant and standoffish.

This type of attitude is also likely to weaken your empathic powers. Truth is multifaceted and always changing. To grasp even a sliver of it, the empath must maintain a balanced connection between their interior and exterior worlds. Shutting either out, or favoring one over the other, will eventually lead the empath to receive misleading messages, or drive them to misinterpret messages that would otherwise be clear and easy to decipher. Empaths are privy to knowledge that often goes unseen, unheard, unacknowledged, but from time to time, they can be flat out wrong--especially if the information they're receiving from the exterior world is limited, it can be skewed to support an incomplete hypothesis.

There is an ancient Indian parable, of possible Buddhist origin, that has become popular in discussions of philosophy and religion, spreading to cultures throughout the world and retold in several different versions, about a group of blind men who encounter an elephant in the jungle. (Perhaps this parable is due for a modern update to include an equal number of blind women--please bear in mind, men are not the only gender susceptible to the pitfalls this proverb warns us.) In this story, each of the blind men must use only their hands to try and comprehend the elephant's size, shape, and overall nature; however, one man's hands find only the elephant's tusks, while another finds only the rough skin of a hind leg, and another still can only feel the animal's full, thin ears. When they compare their experiences, they are each convinced that the others are wrong or insane; in some versions of the story, this inability to agree on their sensory perceptions leads the men to resort to violence. Ultimately, the point of the story, which only the audience can see, is that each of the blind men is right, describing his experience accurately and honestly; the only problem is that they fail to acknowledge the perspectives of others as equally valid.

This is human nature, though the parable aims to inspire us to evolve past it. The truth can never be fully comprehended from one fixed vantage point--it is far too vast for any single person to hold alone. Still, the enlightened empath will be more successful than most at gathering contrasting perspectives and finding a way to incorporate them all into a single philosophy or belief, untangling knots of cognitive dissonance and drawing connections between seemingly disparate concepts--if, and only if, they are willing to stay humble and open to uncomfortable experiences. This pursuit should be handled with care--again, there is a difference between mild discomfort and decisively negative energy, and it's important for the empath to stay guarded against the latter. Don't force yourself to endure an experience that is depleting rather than charging you, but don't let yourself fall into the habit of avoiding the challenging and unpredictable opportunities life offers you, either. As an example, many empaths learn early in their journey to self-empowerment that large crowds can quickly cloud or drain their energy fields; they may have had one particularly difficult or painful experience at a party, concert, funeral, wedding, or rally, and quickly decide that it would be best to avoid large gatherings from that point on. This might be a mistake, though, as joining large groups that are unified in honest intention (a faith-based service, or performance that is effective at steering the emotional path of every audience member, for example) can be one of the most positive and energizing experiences available to the empath.

Though it may be tempting to stay cocooned in whatever emotional spaces feel safest, the empath must make a point of continuously expanding their perspective by trying new things, meeting new people, and seeking out challenges for the sake of growth. The most important thing for an empath to know is just how much the universe has yet to teach them.

Conclusion

Thank you for making it through to the end of Empath: a Survival Guide for the Highly Sensitive Person. Let's hope it has been informative and able to provide you with all of the tools you need to achieve your goals, whatever they may be.

The next steps will vary from one empath to the next. You may want to do further reading on the science of empathy or the insights that the field of clinical psychology can offer. Working with a therapist or counselor can be enormously helpful, allowing you to more quickly process and release emotions that haven't originated within you. If you found the chapter on energy healing to be particularly compelling, you might instead choose to schedule a Reiki initiation with a master or look for a school of modern mysteries to provide further guidance on advanced spiritual practice. It is essen-

Conclusion

tial for empaths with any degree of power to continually monitor their emotional balance, purge negativity, replenish energy, and seek higher clarity and truth. Embrace these practices as part of a lifelong journey, and recognize that even if you ascend to the level of a spiritual teacher or guide for others, there will always be more to learn.

It can also be incredibly healing and inspiring to open your eyes to all the empathic power around you, much of which is still dormant, not yet fully realized or understood. Use the metrics outlined in the second and third chapter of this book, and ask yourself if you might know other empaths who haven't awakened their sensitive powers yet. Or perhaps you know some self-aware empaths that you couldn't recognize as such before now. Whatever the case, you can benefit immensely from expanding your empathic support system. Since empaths are often able to see everything clearly except themselves, let your fellow empaths be a metaphysical mirror. Teach each other, trust each other; heal each other, replenish and amplify each other's energies. You may discover an echelon of both outward love and self-love that you never knew existed before.

While masters and advanced spiritual guides have a great deal of wisdom to share, you should never discount or dismiss the intelligence of your peers, even those who are younger or several steps behind you on the path to self-discovery. One of the most crucial learning skills you can

Conclusion

hone is your ability to unlearn; stay curious, open-minded, and trust in the innate knowledge we are all granted by the universe. Remember, we display powerful empathic connections in infancy, losing touch with our emotional bodies as we grow older and, supposedly, wiser. Do your best to break down the emotional walls you've built inside yourself for the sake of protection; let go of the need for certainty, proof, linear progress, and other ideals we start to cling to in adulthood. Nourish your inner child; allow them to feel valued, respected, and listened to. Remember to hold as much affection and reverence for yourself as you do for others. And whenever you reach a fork in the road of your spiritual journey, choose the path of love.

Finally, if you found this book helpful, a review on Amazon is always appreciated!

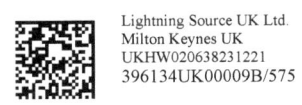